Rapid Weight Loss for Women

Weight loss

Slim down

Rapid weight loss program for women

Your ticket to slim and sexy you

Kate Philips

Introduction

More than 60 percent of Americans aged 20 years and older are overweight.

One-quarter of American adults are also obese.

Globally, there are more than 1 billion overweight adults; at least 300 million of them are obese.

Being obese and overweight puts you at a major risk for chronic diseases, including type 2 diabetes, cardiovascular disease, hypertension and stroke, and certain forms of cancer. And you may already be experiencing some of the signs of chronic illness.

But no matter where you are today, you still have time to take control of your life, get healthy and fit, and stay that way. Get ready to read this book all the way through, and then TAKE ACTION to get rid your life of the things that cause you to be fat, while replacing them with the things that will make you thinner and healthier.

Whenever it comes to undertaking ventures like weight loss, it is extremely imperative to hunt down the perfect method for the reduction of weight. Choose an efficient diet plan. Stay a thousand miles away from the unhealthy diet pills that induce dozens of side effects and all those weight loss supplements on which you stumble upon daily on the internet and television channels, is of critical importance as well. If you could combine a healthy and proper diet with some light workout, they can be the passport for you to the quickest method of cutting down excessive body fats in an absolutely natural way.

The most basic, yet crucial thing to keep in mind is that in order to gain positive results quickly out of any weight loss plan you must neither skip your meals nor eat in an irregular way. If you think that skipping one or two meals, and then having a heavy one once in a day could ever aid in slimming down, then it is nothing but an utter misconception. Additionally, try to ensure that you always set realistic and achievable targets of losing weight before you start following any sort of weight loss plan. Do your best to accomplish the preset goals. Never forget that the human body can only be stretched to a particular limit with the help of a healthy and well balanced meal plan.

Chapter 1

Understanding the Problem

• The Reality of Overweight among Women

The first thing most people mistakenly think when they look at their weight, especially if they are overweight, is that they eat too much. The second thing they mistakenly think is that they eat too much fat, which may be the case, but not all fat is bad for you.

So what is really making you fat?

• The Causes of Overweight

Fast Food

Several aspects of fast food combine to make eating it a detrimental habit. Fast food is, at its core, fast; people become hooked on the convenience of its drive-through or delivery, with negative results in the long term.

And research shows that obesity caused by a fast-food diet is not an isolated problem (which you have probably noticed by looking around at the people eating at these establishments). A USDA report on fast-food consumption states that "three of 10 consumers agreed that meals at a restaurant or fast-food establishment are essential to the way they live," with 75 percent of young people between 11 and 18 eating at fast-food establishments at least 3 times a week.

Combine with those numbers the fact that every day, nearly one-third of U.S. children aged 4 to 19 eat fast food. Which packs on about six extra pounds per child, per year, and increases the risk of obesity, as discovered by a study of 6,212 youngsters.

And if fast food causes children, who generally are more active and have higher metabolisms than adults, to gain 6 pounds a year. Just imagine what it is doing to you!

Why does fast food cause obesity?

Too Many Calories

A typical fast food meal has an energy density of 150% more than an average traditional meal, plus it contains many more calories than a similarly-sized portion of a healthy meal. When these extra calories are consistently consumed, without extra exercise, then the input of calories exceeds the use of calories, and the excess energy provided by the calories is stored as fat.

In the not-so-distant past, this fat storage would have helped us survive lean times. But in the era of cheap, easy to get food, there are rarely lean times that would allow us to lose the weight. So until we evolve, we either have to work off the calories or consume fewer of them.

Unhealthy Ingredients

Fast foods also contain high amounts of sodium (salt), oil, refined sugar, refined flour, and MSG, which are all highly processed and no good for the body. The reason they make you fat are that they contribute to a little discussed cause of obesity: nutrient deficiency. Nutrient deficiencies lead to upset body chemistry, which results in a host of degenerative diseases, as well as weight problems.

Top 5 things in fast food that are disrupting your nutrient levels and making you fat:

Salt- Salt, in itself, is not a bad thing. In fact, you need it to live. The problem is that most of the salt on the market, especially that being used in fast foods and processed foods (most foods that come in a box or can at the grocery store), has been completely stripped of any nutrients.

The second problem is the amount of salt being consumed.

A recent study found that nearly seventy-seven percent of dietary sodium comes from processed foods and restaurants. For example, one McDonald's Quarter Pounder with Cheese has 1,190 mg of sodium, which is basically a whole day's worth. One Extra Crispy Chicken Breast from KFC contains 1,010 mg of sodium, not including the mashed potatoes and gravy and a biscuit, which tacks on an extra 1060 mg of sodium.

And it doesn't stop there. Take a look at your frozen dinners, jarred pasta sauce, canned soup, and almost every packaged food you get at the grocery store. What does it have in common? It is chock full of sodium, along with many other harmful ingredients.

Oil- The oils used in foods, from the buns to the French fries, at fast food restaurants are much different from the healthy oils you get from avocados, coconuts, nuts or fish.

Why?

Many restaurants still use something called partially hydrogenated soybean oil, also known as partially hydrogenated vegetable oil, both of which contain Trans fat. Trans fat has been linked to all kinds of health problems including cancer, type 2 diabetes, decreased immune function and reproductive problems.

Furthermore, while many companies label their products "Trans fat free," the FDA still allows for a little trans fat per serving that does not have to be labeled, and companies are slipping it in under smaller portion sizes.

Even if the soybean oil is fully hydrogenated (it has to be either partially or fully hydrogenated to be used for cooking, but fully hydrogenated is slightly less bad for you), it is high in omega-6 fat. And while we do require some omega-6, most people in the US get way too much, resulting in chronic inflammation, which is the underlying cause of almost all chronic illness like diabetes, cancer, heart disease, etc.

Refined Sugar- Refined sugar is another of those foods that might have been okay for you in a less refined form, but the processing it has undertaken to produce the flavor and look you know as sugar, has stripped it of all beneficial nutrients.

When you eat white sugar, which is listed as an ingredient in nearly every fast food and processed food you eat (along with its evil cousin high-fructose corn syrup). You are actually depleting minerals like calcium, phosphorous, chromium, magnesium, cobalt, copper, zinc, and manganese that help your liver process fats and get them out of your body. In essence, eating white, refined sugar causes your body to pull nutrients from its own bones and tissue in which they are stored, which then causes a wide variety of health problems.

Refined Flour- If you think that the effects of sugar are bad on your body, then you may be surprised to learn that white, refined flour is even worse. It is nutritionally deadly, and if you tried to live on bread alone for 60 days, you would die of malnutrition.

The reason is that when white flour is made, the healthy parts, including the wheat kernel, wheat germ, and wheat oil, which contain important things like B vitamins and over 100 other vitamins and fibers that help you digest the wheat, are all taken out.

Finally, white flour has been bleached in a process that produces a chemical called alloxan. Alloxan has been proven to cause diabetes by destroying the beta cells in a human pancreas.

MSG (Monosodium Glutamate)- MSG, also known as monosodium glutamate, may be one of the most deadly food additives on the market. It replaces salt in many processed foods and fast foods for a very good reason: it is addictive.

Not only does it enhance the flavor of food, but it is also anexcitotoxin, which means that it overexcites the cells in your brain to the point of cell damage or death and causes brain damage to varying degrees. Eating MSG can trigger learning disabilities, Alzheimer's disease, Parkinson's disease, Lou Gehrig's disease, and MS.

And that's not all! To make Trans fat, scientists inject them with MSG. Injecting a baby rat with 2 to 4 milligrams of MSG per kilogram of body weight can turn a healthy rat into an obese, addictive, insulin resistant or diabetic rat in just 5 days.

The worst part is that MSG is in almost every packaged food and fast food including fries, any breaded and fried chicken, special or secret sauces, sausage, dressings, soups, cheeses, pizza sauce, Alfredo sauce, anything with soy sauce, meat tenderizers and marinades and more.

And MSG is not only listed under one name. Many restaurants and food manufacturers advertise that their food is MSG free, but the MSG is actually just listed under another name including the ones below:

Autolyzed yeast

Calcium casein ate

Gelatin

Glutamate

Glutamic acid

Hydrolyzed protein

Monopotassium glutamate

Sodium casein ate

Textured protein

Yeast extract

Yeast food

Yeast nutrient

Just keep in mind that, just because it is under a different name, does not mean that MSG is any less potent, or any better for you.

Soft Drinks

Carbonated soft drinks are the single largest source of calories in the North American diet, accounting for about 7 percent of our daily calories. According to the Center for Science in the Public Interest, teenagers get 13 percent of their calories from soft drinks, and the average American drinks up to 50 gallons of soft drinks annually!

Soft drinks have been named as one of the leading causes of being overweight and obesity-along with Type 2 diabetes and other weight-related illnesses. They contain high-fructose corn syrup (HFCS), which is toxic to the body, in particular the liver, because the liver cannot process it efficiently.

But don't think you are off the hook if you drink only diet sodas. Diet sodas contain an artificial sweetener known as aspartame, which a group of researchers at Purdue University found to cause weight gain in those who consume it regularly.

They reported that artificial sweeteners, like aspartame, trick the body into thinking it is consuming sugar, which causes the release of insulin. The problem is that the insulin is not really needed, and the excess of it in the bloodstream can lead to metabolic confusion and cause you to pack on the pounds.

Incorrect Food Combinations

According to food combination experts, one of the worst things we can do to our digestive system is combine starches and proteins in the same meal. That means the All-American meal of meat and potatoes is actually bad for us!

Proteins and starches both need a specific digestive environment in order to be digested well. Proteins digest best when the acid levels of the stomach are higher, while starches digest best when the alkaline levels are higher.

When proteins and starches cannot be properly digested, it leads to improper absorption. Improper absorption, in turn, can lead to a number of different digestive and health problems such as indigestion, bloating, gas, fatigue, high cholesterol, and weight gain.

Therefore, it is important to eat your proteins and your starches at separate meals, with at least 2-3 hours between them for digestion.

Here is a sample daily eating schedule:

Breakfast - Omelet w/ Vegetables or Meat

Snack- Granola bar or Fruit or Cereal

Lunch- Salad w/ Chicken or Tuna

Snack- Crackers or Yogurt or Pretzels

Dinner - Chicken, Meat, or Fish & Vegetable

Snack- Popcorn or Fruit

Stress & Depression

Lead author, Paula Rhode, PhD, a clinical psychologist and professor of preventative medicine and public health at the University of Kansas, mentioned that increasing levels of stress accurately predicted increased body mass index (BMI), increased weight gain, increased caloric intake, and higher dietary fat intake. She found that stress and depression predicted 26% of the variance in weight gain and 29% of the increase in BMI.

The reason that stress causes us to gain weight is simple. Our body, specifically our neuroendocrine system, is wired to help us survive. To our ancestors, stress may have been an attacking wild animal, while today it might be our job or bills. However, our neuroendocrine system does not know the difference, and it activates a series of hormones whenever we feel stressed.

These hormones are present to help us fight or flee whatever is stressing us. They include, adrenalin, which gives us a sudden burst of energy, corticotrophin, and cortisol, which is the main hormone that causes belly fat.

Cortisol works to help us replenish our body after the stress or threat has passed, and in elevated levels, it makes us feel hungry, driving us to eat. The problem is that we, most likely, have not had to literally fight or flee from our stress, so we haven't had to expend our energy to avert the danger.

Instead, we sit and stew in our frustration or worry, and eat to feel better and to reduce our cortisol back to normal levels, thus eating extra calories and gaining weight at each instance of stress. And in this day and age, that can be quite often!

The Lifestyle Problem that Lead to Obesity

According to a poll of nearly 6,300 people, by the Institute for Medicine and Public Health, it's likely that you spend a stunning 56 hours a week planted like a geranium-staring at your computer screen, working the steering wheel, or collapsed in a heap in front of your high-definition TV. And it turns out that women may be more sedentary than men, since they tend to play fewer sports and hold less active jobs.

When you sit for an extended period of time, your body starts to shut down at the metabolic level, says Marc Hamilton, Ph.D., associate professor of biomedical sciences at the University of Missouri. And when our metabolism slows, but we continue to eat, often more out of habit than actual hunger, we consume too many calories and gain weight. In particular, a slow metabolism equals more abdominal fat.

Television Viewing

According to a National Health and Nutrition Examination survey, 65% of American adults over 20 years of age are overweight. 30% are obese, and 5% extremely obese. For African Americans, the prevalence of obesity is even higher. Among black women over 20 years of age, 77% are overweight, and 49% are obese.

And while those numbers are disturbing, researchers believe there may be a link: then average American spends 34 hours watching TV every week, plus another 3-6 hours watching pre-recorded shows or movies. Add that to the amount of time sitting at work, and there is no wonder we are a culture of overweight people.

A recent body of research proposed three not-so-surprising links between obesity and TV viewing:

TV viewing replaces outdoor activities and exercises.

TV leads to excessive food consumption while watching.

Exposure to advertisements in TV prime time programming leads to subsequent consumption of advertised foods.

Furthermore, it is no secret that prolonged inactivity can slow your metabolism, meaning that your body becomes stuck in a rut of collecting fat, rather than using the calories you consume.

Hormonal imbalance

There are a number of hormone disorders that can cause weight gain and chronic inability to lose weight. The most common syndromes include growth hormone deficiency, Cushing's syndrome, and hypothyroidism.

Each syndrome has its own unique features and rarely is weight gain the only symptom. For example, growth hormone deficiency is associated with short stature, thin and dry skin, and low muscle mass and mainly abdominal body fat. Cushing's syndrome can lead to sweating, high blood pressure, depression, anxiety, and stretch marks. Hypothyroidism often causes mental slowing, intolerance to cold, fatigue, and constipation.

If you are obese or very overweight, and you have trouble losing weight with proper diet and regular exercise, and you have any of the symptoms listed above, you may want to get tested for hormonal imbalance. It is important to seek help because you are at higher risk for diabetes, heart disease and many other medical problems.

Furthermore, keeping on extra pounds, no matter what their cause, can not only affect your appearance and your self-image, but it can also put you at risk for many chronic and life-shortening diseases. In the next section, I will give you a no-nonsense plan for losing weight and keeping it off, even if you have failed at dieting before.

Checklist No. 1

1. Do you have an obesity problems?

A. Yes

B. Somewhat

C. Unsure

D. Not at all

2. Do you love to eat fast food?

A. Yes

B. Somewhat

C. Unsure

D. Not at all

3. Do you love to eat salty foods or foods that have a lot of preservatives like MSG (monosodium glutamate)?

A. Yes

B. Somewhat

C. Unsure

D. Not at all

4. Are you fond of drinking soft drinks?

A. Yes

B. Somewhat

C. Unsure

D. Not at all

5. Are you living a stressful life that often lead to depression?

A. Yes

B. Somewhat

C. Unsure

D. Not at all

6. Are you suffering from any health problems related to obesity?

A. Yes

B. Somewhat

C. Unsure

D. Not at all

7. Do you have a sedentary lifestyle?

A. Yes

B. Somewhat

C. Unsure

D. Not at all

Chapter 2: Understanding the Basics

The Truth about Calorie Intake

If you are trying to lose weight faster, the one word that won't escape your ears is "calorie." You will find it in every diet you can think of and it will also be present in every exercise. If this is your first time hearing this word, go easy on yourself if you don't comprehend the reason it is so popular.

In essence, a calorie is just a unit of heat energy; it is what gives you power after you eat. Without it, you would find it impossible to perform any activity. Think of it in this way: calories are like fuel for the body. Without them, life would cease to exist. And you certainly would not be reading this now.

Calories come from the food that we eat. Specifically, these are fats, carbohydrates, and proteins.

However, one thing that must be made clear is that a calorie is not a calorie. For example, for every gram of fat, you get 9 calories. But when it comes to carbohydrates and proteins, you obtain 4 calories per gram.

How Do Calories Affect Weight

It does not matter what food you eat or how much you eat, but if your plate is full of food that is high in calories, you are bound to gain weight.

In older to lose 1 pound of fat, you must use 3500 calories (that's the number of calories it takes to make 1 pound). So reducing them in your diet is the only guaranteed way to see the pounds drop on the scale.

If you eat 2500 calories daily, you can lower them to 2000. Assuming that your body uses 2500 calories per day, it means you will have a deficit of 500 calories. So your body will turn to stored fat for energy. By the end of 7 days, 500 calorie-deficits will add up to 3500 calories. So you will lose 1 pound of weight.

However, know that cutting food intake is not the only way to reduce calories. You can also introduce physical activity in your life. So if you can burn an extra 500 calories with exercise, you will have a 1000-calorie deficit daily. In 7 days, it will turn to 7000 calories meaning you will lose 2 pounds of weight in a week.

Checklist No. 2

1. Do you have any idea of what your average calorie intake is?

A. Yes

B. Somewhat

C. Unsure

D. Not at all

2. Do you monitor your calorie intake?

A. Yes

B. Somewhat

C. Unsure

D. Not at all

3. Do you know that your calorie intake affects your weight?

A. Yes

B. Somewhat

C. Unsure

D. Not at all

4. Do you usually cut your calorie intake?

A. Yes

B. Somewhat

C. Unsure

D. Not at all

5. Do you consciously regulate your calorie intake?

A. Yes

B. Somewhat

C. Unsure

D. Not at all

6. Are you aware that reducing your food intake does not ensure your losing weight?

A. Yes

B. Somewhat

C. Unsure

D. Not at all

7. Do you have any idea what the ideal calorie intake every day is?

A. Yes

B. Somewhat

C. Unsure

D. Not at all

Chapter 3:

Understanding the Proper Diet Plans for losing weight effectively

Understanding the Balance Diet

These days, the most commonly followed and highly effective method on which thousands of folks from all over the globe are relying on is the 7-day weight loss meal plan. It is pretty much safe to say that this particular program of coping with the corpulence is simply the best one could ever come across that will show amazing results in the time span of only seven days. This in an absolutely natural way without having to consume diet pills or health supplements. Another great thing about this quickest meal plan for losing weight is that it has been found extremely successful and effective in individuals of both genders as well as of all the age groups. Plus, quite a lot of claims have already been made that people managed to lose around twenty pounds of weight merely within the timeframe of seven days by following this incredible program.

In every part of the mother earth, there are literally tens and thousands of folks who're a little bit chubbier for their personal liking, hence, trying to find diverse ways to get their selves in a good shape without actually investing in loads of effort. There are so many individuals who have been trying a whole plethora of options. Such as regular workout, jogging, running, exercising in a gym and practicing yoga. Some for months, or even years in order to reduce their weight, but could not find success in achieving their goal. If you think you are chubbier and want to do something about it, then you must give a shot to this weight loss meal plan to shed off all your excessive fat deposits.

What Food to Eat

Proteins

Protein is one of the most important nutrients you need for a healthy life. However, this nutrient also helps in weight loss as it makes you feel full for longer. It suppresses your appetite thereby reducing any chances of reaching for other unhealthy food during the day.

Additionally, research has proved that protein is a useful ingredient in the process of fat burning.

Foods that provide this nutrient are many, however, you should ensure that you are only getting it from healthy sources; losing weight does not mean you must endanger your life with unhealthy food. Some examples of foods you can eat to get protein include eggs, beans, fish, lean meat, milk, etc.

Fats

Fat has been demonized for a long time. And I would not blame you if you have been avoiding this nutrient since you realized that you needed to lose weight. However, the truth is that not all types of fats are bad. There are some, actually, that are healthy and you cannot live without. Specifically, I'm referring to unsaturated fats.

It is their saturated counterparts you need to avoid.

Fats take longer to be digested, and so, keep your hunger at bay. Good sources include olive oil, canola oil, almonds, peanut butter, avocados, salmon, walnuts, and other foods.

Carbohydrates

Carbohydrates are also important in your life. In fact, they are food for the brain. You must, however, limit their consumption if you are serious about losing weight. A daily intake of 20-50 grams is all you need to stay alive.

The problem is that carbohydrates are easily digested. This raises your blood sugar level which can be toxic if left unchecked. To prevent the situation reaching poisonous levels, the pancreases releases insulin to clean all the sugar.

Unfortunately, the presence of too much insulin in the blood stops the body from burning fats. And if you stay in this condition frequently, you can bet that you will break the scale the next time you get on it.

Fiber

Fiber is your best friend if you want to lose weight. It fills you up thereby increasing your satiety. Additionally, as it is not easily digestible, it slows the absorption of sugar into the blood. So you do not get hungry soon after eating.

Even better, you can eat as much fibrous food as you need and you will not gain weight because most fiber foods are low in calories. If you know you don't get enough fiber in your diet, start eating these foods: cabbage, broccoli, lettuce, kale, spinach, celery, and other vegetables.

So as you can see, this chapter recommends that you should eat a lot of proteins and fiber. Fats must be included in your diet but in moderate quantities. As for carbohydrates, you must limit their consumption. By eating this way, you should be able to see the pounds drop.

But remember it's calories that make you fat. So make sure that you are keeping track on a number of calories in your diet. Don't forget the rule that to lose weight, you must use more calories than you consume.

Understanding the Needs of your Body

All of us want to be slim & sexy, and there are plenty of products on the market that promise massive fat loss in as little as three days. But face it, nothing other than surgery can help you in such a short time-- at least with any kind of lasting effects.

Most of the lose fat fast schemes are comprised of fad diets or body masks that cause you to lose only the water in your body. Our body is comprised of about 40-60% water, which, when lost, will decrease body weight and maybe even make us look slimmer. But the problem is that these types of diets are neither permanent, nor healthy. The only true and lasting way to lose weight and keep it off is through a change to a healthier lifestyle.

Before, you start imagining your dream body type; you need to identify your body type. In the next section we will discuss various body shapes, how to calculate your body fat percentage, and how to set a realistic weight goal.

Identify Your Body Type

Weight loss depends not only on the weight loss program you are following, but also on your body type and genetics.

If you come from a family where obesity is a serious issue, and you want to look like a skinny lingerie model, I would recommend that you go for surgery and nothing else.

On the other hand, if you are aware of your limitations as a person and the limitations of your genetic potential, this eBook can help you achieve your target.

Again, by target, I do not mean you should think that because you had a 17 inch waist when you were 14, that you can achieve it at the age of 35. You might, but chances are higher that you will not, and it is probably for your own good too! In fact, if you have a broader pelvic region, however hard you try, you might get stuck at a certain waist size and find it very difficult to slim down more. The point is not to push it beyond the edge, and to remember that we want to look *our* best, and become healthier, not just look like a model in a magazine.

A very important thing to understand is the fact that though our bodies function similarly, we need to respect the minute differences. While some people get fat because of overeating, others gain weight because of under eating. Respect yourself for who you are. Before you jump in to any routine exercises, it is in your own interest to know your body type.

Here are typical features for various Body Types:

Ectomorphs

Women who are long, lean and lanky, with a small, delicate bone structure, narrow hips and a small waist are called ectomorphs. Their legs tend to be longer than their torso

Mesomorphs

Mesomorphs tend to be athletic and have broad shoulders and hips, narrow waists and a high percentage of muscle in comparison to fat. These are the "pear-shaped" women.

Endomorphs

Women who are more heavily boned, carry more fat than muscle and accumulate their fat mainly around their abdomens are called endomorphs or apple shaped

If, however, you cannot place yourself in any of the categories, do not worry. Most people have characteristics of two or even all three of the body types.

Body fat measurement – know where you stand with your weight

Obesity is determined **NOT** only by body weight, but also by the measurement of body fat, or your body fat percentage. People might be normal or underweight, but may have excessive body fat. On the other hand, some might be overweight by normal standards, but if they have low body fat, they are not obese.

How to Calculate Body Fat?

Your approximate body fat percentage (%) can be calculated according to the following formula:

Body Fat Percentage = (Body Fat Weight x 100) / total bodyweight

Body Fat Weight = Total bodyweight - Lean Body Mass

Lean Body Mass = A + B + E - C –D

You can find the values of A, B, C, D, and E from the following:

For Women:

A = (Total body weight x 0.732) + 8.987

B = Wrist measurement (at fullest point) / 3.140

C = Waist measurement (at naval) x 0.157

D = Hip measurement (at fullest point) x 0.249

E = Forearm measurement (at fullest point) x 0.434

An ideal fat percentage for females should be between 18%-20% of your total body weight. So anything over that means that you do need to lose weight or more precisely, fat.

Just remember to consider that "weight" consists of both lean body mass and body fat. And your goal is to lose the fat while creating more muscle, so while your fat percentage may decrease over time, your weight may go up or down only slightly. That does not mean that you are not reaching your healthy lifestyle goals.

Try to keep your weight loss goals realistic, and remember, keep the calorie-burning muscle, and lose only the fat.

How to Get the Perfect Body?

Is there such a thing as the perfect female body and if so, should you be attempting to achieve it?

I believe there is a perfect female body and the closer you approach that ideal, the closer you will be to health and attractiveness.

Evolutionary research shows that a WHR (waist to hip ratio) of 0.7 and a WBR (waist-to-breast ratio) of 0.7 are considered to be ideal. The 36-24-36 ideal results in a curvaceously thin female with small waist and hips and large breasts. This is very difficult to achieve naturally, and you should instead focus on the above ratios for a healthier, slim body.

What It Means To Have A Fit Body?

Physical fitness and healthy body both are important. We can characterize physical fitness as:

Fat-to-Muscle Ratio - the amount of fat percentage you carry to the lean muscle percentage. A higher ratio of muscle is more desirable for a healthy, fit body.

Muscle Fat and Flexibility - pertains to the strength and flexibility of your muscles, bones, ligaments and tendons that aid in easy movement. Fitness level of your body determines by the strength and flexibility of your muscle.

Cardiovascular Endurance- the relationship that your heart shares with the rest of the transport systems. A better cardiovascular endurance ensures that all your body's muscles are supplied with enough nutrients and oxygen. It helps you to climb a flight of stairs at one go or to run and play around with your kids.

Absolute vs Relative Deficit

The part in understanding the needs of your body include knowing the absolute deficit against relative deficit. Absolute deficit means the deficit in our body like the essential nutrients that your body needs to be replenish. Proteins, carbohydrates and essential fats are the essential nutrients that often needs to be replenish for proper functioning of your body.

While relative deficit are deficits in our body like the nutrients that usually are satisfied when you are eating balance diet. They are usually met in small amounts and need not to be satisfied in huge amount. Vitamins and micronutrients like minerals are usually present in the food we eat. Often times we think that these things need to be supplied in an amount that it usually required. This often causes us unnecessary food intake thus causing overweight issues especially in women.

Checklist No. 3

1. Do you eat a well-balanced diet?

A. Yes

B. Somewhat

C. Unsure

D. Not at all

2. Do you know what body type do you have?

A. Yes

B. Somewhat

C. Unsure

D. Not at all

3. Are you aware that your weight depends on your body type?

A. Yes

B. Somewhat

C. Unsure

D. Not at all

4. Are you aware that body mass index and fat body index are important in determining what type of diet you have to use?

A. Yes

B. Somewhat

C. Unsure

D. Not at all

5. Do you know how to compute your body and fat mass index?

A. Yes

B. Somewhat

C. Unsure

D. Not at all

6. Do you understand how to be truly body fit?

A. Yes

B. Somewhat

C. Unsure

D. Not at all

7. Do you understand what the difference between absolute and relative deficit is?

A. Yes

B. Somewhat

C. Unsure

D. Not at all

Chapter 4:

Different Diet Plans

Paleo Diet

What is the Paleo Diet?

The Paleo diet has other popular names such as "the cave-man diet", and "the Paleolithic or Stone-Age diet". These names clearly explain what it's all about. The Paleo diet is all about eating the way our ancestors did way back. Those brave men and strong women lived without all that comfort we have now and without all these foods that make us fat or do not provide the necessary vitamins for healthy living. We are talking about the foods that hunters-gatherers ate, not farmers who are able to grow food because of the developments in agriculture. While many people turn to vegan diets discovering that they don't get everything that their bodies require, the Paleo diet is a healthy way to keep off excess weight and to address many health issues ensuring that you get what your body needs.

This diet ensures a high intake of vitamins, antioxidants, protein, minerals, fiber, potassium and healthy fats, such as Omega 3 and a low sodium and carbohydrate intake. Basically it means that your diet will include exactly what you need and exclude what is not necessary for your body, mind and wellness in general.

Many people nowadays have health and especially weight issues because they are lactose and gluten intolerant. This diet is free of both lactose and gluten. Your diet will consist of fruits, vegetables, meat, healthy oils, seafood, eggs, roots and seeds and great variety of natural spices, but you will exclude dairy products, refined sugar, grains and cereals, refined vegetable oils, potatoes, legumes like peanuts, beans, peas and lentils, pasta and unhealthy processed foods. It's not as difficult as it might sound at the beginning. Once you start with the Paleo diet, you will definitely feel a lot better and will therefore not think about giving it up. The Paleo diet requires only one thing from you: knowledge of what you're eating. This means that you acknowledge what actually allows your body to function properly and what is tasty, healthy food.

You might have heard that eating red meat can increase the chance of getting cancer or heart disease. Well, modern science has something else to say: get rid of these beliefs. Cooking red meat in an improper way really might harm your health, for example, if you cook it in a pan with a lot of salt and refined vegetable oil or butter. So, yes, that's the key: the preparation of your food!

One more enjoyable fact is that the Paleo diet is neither too fat, nor tasteless, nor does it require that you live without the tastes that you love. Eradicating sugar from your meals does not mean that you won't get sweet tastes through the food you eat in the Paleo diet. In the same way, no longer consuming dairy products does not mean that you won't get enough of calcium, because there are many other and a lot healthier products that will provide you with the necessary amount of calcium. We will talk more about products ideal for the Paleo diet in the following chapters.

Oh, and if you like to exercise, the Paleo diet ensures that your workouts are a lot more effective! It means that the same exercise that you do, even the simplest form of exercise, such as those daily actions that include taking stairs, walking or gardening in your backyard, will bring far better results!

What about you're eating schedule and how to fit it in with your agenda? It's easy: you eat when you want to eat. Cavemen did not eat after looking at the clock – they ate when they wanted to eat.

Cavemen also didn't count calories. If you feel happier doing so, feel free to count them; you will find the calorie count for each recipe here in this book, but remember that your body actually tells you how much you need if you stick to healthy food. The Paleo diet is nutritious and fulfilling enough to keep you away from storing unwanted fat in your body.

What is slow cooking?

The Paleo diet includes a lot of tasty raw foods, but you might already know how to deal with these – wash, cut and eat. This, however, does not mean that you'll only be able to eat cold foods. It's not just healthy, but truly tasty as well, and most of the recipes do not require that you stand staring at the food while it's cooking and stirring it every 3 minutes.

Slow cooking means simmering and preparing food on relatively low temperatures – a very gentle method in which to cook food. The catch as to why slow cooking is so much healthier than other cooking methods is that it makes food a lot more tender and the nutrient content of vegetables does not decrease as much as it does when cooking food outwit a slow cooker. The Paleo diet food cooked in a slow cooker does not lose as many vitamins in comparison to fast cooking on a high heat and along with that, the flavors of the ingredients you use mix well in a slow cooker so you get to experience new and enjoyable tastes. What slow cooking really means is less time on preparation and more on cooking to make sure that you gain as much as possible from your food. One more very important thing is that slow cooking is absolutely great for preparing large amounts of food: a slow cooker cooks large pieces of meat thoroughly while you are working out, while you are at work or on your way to collect children from school. Slow cooking ensures that your life doesn't stop to prepare meals.

Paleo diet and slow cooking are the perfect match

One thing that scares many people is that slow cooking means you can't just run into your kitchen, drop whatever you have in the refrigerator into a pan, and eat it within a few minutes. This shouldn't be something that you're worrying about: the Paleo diet doesn't mean that whatever you have from now on you will only prepare in your slow cooker. Meals are as easy and convenient as putting all the ingredients into one pot and then leaving! Return after few hours and enjoy your meal, or have your food ready to reheat and enjoy later on! In fact, the Paleo diet and slow cooking are a match made in heaven and here's why:

It's healthy (you already know this);

It's easy and you do not need to be an amazing chef to achieve delicious results;

Slow cooking your Paleo diet food is a way to prepare your food for more than just one day or one person;

You can do whatever you wish as your slow cooker does the work for you because your food doesn't require attention while it's cooking;

You will discover more natural tastes;

You can prepare large pieces of meat without overdoing them and/or drying out the meat;

When you come home from work, a freshly cooked, healthy, warm meal is there waiting for you;

You can make many different dishes using the same ingredients that can be found easily, for example, carrots;

The meals are so nutritious that you are naturally kept away from overeating, and, as a consequence, gaining weight and causing health problems;

Your energy levels increase and this therefore helps you to lose excess weight;

Paleo slow cooking provides you with different kinds of healthy foods: warm, cold, tender, spicy, mild, bite-sized, light, hearty, and large amounts of food cooked thoroughly; and

You'll maintain your shape without too much effort.

How slow cooking saves you time and money

Electric crock-pots for slow cooking are not too expensive, and they are absolutely safe to leave them plugged into electricity for a long period of time while you are not around.

A slow-cooker uses electricity and saves you money as it doesn't use more electric power than a light bulb.

You are not required to spend a lot to vary your meals and there is no need for you to buy expensive ingredients to experience new tastes. Slow cooking does the job of bringing out new flavors for you.

You will save money that you previously spent on unhealthy, processed foods. Following your old diet, you would have also had to have spent more money on restoring your health in an attempt to repair the damage you may have caused.

Slow cooking asks for a few minutes of your time to prepare the ingredients and that's it. While the food is cooking, you are free to do whatever you need to do. If time is money, a slow-cooker provides you with that.

A slow cooker enables you to make delicious food using readily available and cheap ingredients, such as vegetables. Cheap can taste just as great if you give it a try and simmer it in a slow cooker.

Slow cooking saves your time and money because you cut expenses on solving health issues – this diet keeps you healthy.

What you need – equipment

The main thing here is a slow cooker or a crock-pot - an electronic device with a ceramic bowl and lid. Crock-pots are really easy to use, you can regulate the heat and cooking time, and it's safe to leave them for long time when you're not at home. Using a crock-pot honestly makes life a lot easier.

If you do not have an electric slow-cooker just yet, there are alternatives you can use in which you can steam and simmer foods on a low heat:

Dutch oven – a pot with tight walls and a lid. You will obtain the best results by placing it in the oven.

Casserole dish – a deep saucepan to cook food, again in the oven.

Regular (oven-proof) pot – you can heat this either in oven or on low-heat on your gas or electric stove, but you will have to stir it from time to time so that the food doesn't stick to the walls of the pot or burn the bottom of the pot.

With these alternatives in mind, you can still achieve the same delicious results as if you were using an electric device, but some dishes just might ask for some more attention during the cooking process.

For some dishes, you will need a pan to brown the ingredients to obtain some different flavors and to maintain consistency before putting them into the electric slow cooker (or its alternatives).

Some other recipes call for foil or parchment paper to place in the slow cooker, of for you to use a blender, food processor, or toothpicks.

Other pieces of equipment that you require are every day kitchen items such as a knife, fork, grater, etc.

What you need – products

Here's a quick reminder of products that you definitely won't need and that **are NOT used in a Paleo diet**:

Sugar: this means any kind of brown, white or other refined sugar and candy. Alternatives to refined sugars that are used in the Paleo diet are maple syrup or honey, but remember, you use these in small doses and they are not for everyday use.

Legumes: beans, peas, lentils and peanuts.

Grains: corn, wheat, barley, oatmeal, rye, rice and others. It means that you will have to exclude flour and also products such as muffins, pancakes, pizza, pasta and bread. You will, however, learn how to make bread without using grain flour in this book.

Starch vegetables: yams and potatoes are a no-no, although many people support using sweet potatoes in a Paleo diet. And, yes, you really don't need potato chips to be healthy in life!

Dairy products: milk, all kinds of cheese, butter and yoghurt, cream and ice-cream. Stone-age people used milk only to feed infants, and they didn't acquire milk from any species of animal. Milk is really only necessary for infants and even they don't drink milk from other species when a mother breastfeeds, right?

Salt: salted fish and meat products such as salami, etc. are not allowed. You won't feel as though you're missing out on salt though because the Paleo diet offers its own alternative to refined salt, and that is sea salt.

And add to this list all artificially sweetened fruit and berry juices, ketchup, mayonnaise, soft drinks and soda drinks from the supermarket shelves because they are packed with sugar and preservatives that your body has no need for.

Don't be worried! The list of what you CAN eat is a lot longer!

This is what a healthy, delicious, and nutritious Paleo diet advises you to **include in your menu**:

- **Meat:** beef, pork, turkey, duck, chicken and other poultry; lamb, goat, and rabbit. When purchasing meat, the best option is always grass-fed meat and if you're one to worry about calories and fat, you should trim off any excess fat. As long as the meat you buy is not processed in an unhealthy way with added artificial preservatives, it has a place on your table. Organ meat such as tongue, kidney, liver, heart and marrow are welcome as well!

- **Seafood, fish and shellfish**: salmon, tuna, herring, eel, trout, mackerel, crab, mussels, lobster, oysters, shrimp, octopus, squid, shark, swordfish, roe and others are all great, just make sure that you buy your seafood products from a safe source and avoid all canned fish meat.

- **Mushrooms:** cremini, Portobello, shiitake, bolete, chanterelle, rehash, mistake, porcini and other mushrooms are all fine for you to eat.

- **Fruits, vegetables and leafy greens:** apples, apricots, kiwis, lemons, mangos, melons, nectarines, pears, oranges, pineapples, watermelon, grapefruit, avocados, arugula, artichokes, different kinds of peppers, tomatoes, pumpkins, rhubarb, squashes, asparagus, broccoli, Brussels sprouts, cabbage, endives, grapes, leeks, olives, cauliflower, cucumber, eggplant, onion greens, spinach, zucchini, etc. The list is endless. The main thing is to ensure that you buy these foods unprocessed. Do take into account that buying raisins, dried plums, apricots or other dried fruits may contain a lot of added sugar. If you are buying dried fruits or berries, make sure there is no added sugar in them! Plums and raisins are naturally sweet enough that you can use them to satisfy any cravings for sugar. These food products actually do not require any refined sugar added to them.

- **Berries:** strawberries, cherries, blackberries, blueberries, blackcurrants, cranberries, etc.

- **Roots:** carrots, garlic and different kinds of onions, radishes, celery, turnips, ginger, horseradish, parsnips and so on.

- **Nuts and seeds** (that you can easily gather from nature without cultivation): almonds, pine nuts, walnuts, hazelnuts, cashew nuts, coconuts, pecans, macadamia nuts, pistachios and other nuts; pumpkin seeds, sunflower seeds, and sesame seeds. These nuts and seeds are truly healthy, but just make sure that you don't eat packs and packs of them and avoid buying any salted or roasted nuts and seeds! Peanuts are not on this list because they are in fact legumes and not nuts.

- **Herbs and spices:** parsley, cilantro, dill, basil, grated pepper, cinnamon, bay leaves, coriander, cloves, rosemary, cumin, marjoram, oregano, peppermint, thyme, cardamom, mustard and a lot more. In place of refined salt, use sea salt!

- **Oils** (for salads and cooking): avoid refined vegetable oils because there are a lot of far healthier alternatives available that go well with a Paleo diet such as olive, almond, coconut, avocado, sesame seed or walnut oils.

- **Eggs**

- **Drinks:** drinks suitable for this diet include water, freshly squeezed juices without added sugar, coconut milk, almond milk, coffee and tea (without sugar or sweeteners!) and smoothies.

- **Refined sugar substitutes:** raw honey, organic maple syrup, organic apple sauce, dried raisins and dates (without added preservatives), coconut sugar, ripe bananas, and agave nectar. .

- **Refined salt substitutes:** sea salt

- **Milk substitutes:** cashew milk, coconut milk, and almond milk.

- **Butter substitutes:** coconut oil (it has a solid consistency in room temperature and lower, but melts when heated, just like butter), mashed avocado (if not for greasing pots and pans), and almond butter.

So, to summarize the list of Paleo diet foods, always remember that if something can be gathered or hunted and if cavemen could eat it without using an agricultural means of growing, you can include it in your menu as well. Of course, we live in the21st century, and so this does mean that products, such as a glass of wine, won't hurt to drink, but **keep your use of these kinds of beverages in moderation.** These are further food products and beverages whose usage you should keep in check: wine, beer, tea, coffee, sweetening with honey or maple syrup; avoid eating too many nuts, dried fruits and berries and avoid using too much oil. Even if something is healthy, you should still keep a count of how often you are consuming these foods and beverages, simply add them to your meals from time to time, but avoid making them the main ingredient in a dish by placing them at the centre of your meal every day and you will be totally fine!

Dash Diet

The DASH diet is a well-balanced, lifelong approach to healthy eating that was discovered in research funded by the National Institutes of Health (NIH) to determine the role of dietary eating patterns on blood pressure.

Over the years a number of studies have proven that the DASH diet is not only effective for lowering blood pressure through diet. It is also effective in reducing the risk of cardiovascular disease, several types of cancers, stroke, heart disease, kidney stones, kidney disease, diabetes, heart failure and many other diseases. The DASH diet has also been shown to promote weight loss and improve overall health.

The Dash diet is recommended by:

The Mayo Clinic

That American Heart Association

The American College of Cardiology

The Dietary Guidelines for Americans

US guidelines for the treatment of hypertension

The National Heart, Lung and Blood Institute (a part of the National Institutes of Health [NIH] of the US Department of Health & Human Services)

The best overall diet

In January 2014 US News and World Report selected the DASH diet as the best overall diet, the healthiest diet and the best diet for diabetes for four years in a row.

The DASH diet was chosen by a distinguished panel of doctors for its healthy balance of food groups, its ability to improve health and its proven track record of successfully working time and time again.

Why was the Dash Diet Created?

DASH stands for **D**ietary Approaches to **S**top **H**ypertension. Hypertension or high blood pressure has been on the rise in the US for the past 50 years.

The continued increase of hypertension led the National Institutes of Health to propose funding for research that would study the impact of dietary patterns on blood pressure.

In 1992, the National Heart, Lung and Blood Institute worked closely with five prestigious medical research centers in the US to design and carry out the largest and most detailed study ever conducted called "The DASH study."

The DASH study was uniquely based on foods that the average person could buy at a local grocery store thus making it easy for anyone to implement.

The DASH Diet and Weight Loss

Although the DASH diet was not formally created as a weight loss diet it does promote weight loss. This is due to the DASH diets food groups and guidelines.

The well balanced blend of nutritious low calorie whole foods helps your body drop unnecessary weight.

There are three things about the DASH diet that make it particularly great for **weight loss**:

Consuming healthy fats and omitting unhealthy fats

High fiber intake

High vitamin C intake

The DASH diet and fats

The average American diet contains a lot of unhealthy fat. Trans fats and saturated fats are extremely unhealthy, high in calories and have low to no nutritional value. They are the number one cause of weight gain on the Standard American Diet (SAD diet). These fats are extremely limited on the DASH diet.

Healthy plant-based fats and omega-3 fatty acids on the other hand are an important part of the DASH diet and highly encouraged. Good fats are excellent for the body and the waist line!

The DASH diet and fiber

The DASH diet includes a lot of foods that contain soluble and insoluble fiber. A high fiber diet helps you feel full longer, slows the absorption of dietary fiber and sugar in your body and improves digestion.

This prevents blood sugar spikes while minimizing carbohydrate and junk food cravings. It also prevents fat from being stored in the abdominal area.

A high fiber diet is excellent for your overall health and weight loss!

The DASH diet and Vitamin C

The DASH diet encourages a high consumption of fresh fruits and vegetables that are full of vitamins, minerals and antioxidants. One vitamin that plays a huge role in weight loss is vitamin C.

Vitamin C aids in the elimination of stored fat and it prevents hormonal reactions from occurring that can promote fat storage in the abdomen.

Problem is, vitamin C is easily depleted. Stress is the number one thing that depletes vitamin C. When your body is lacking vitamin C it tells your brain that you're under stress. This causes a release of the stress hormone cortisol that is sent out to store fat in the abdomen as a safety measure against the threat of famine.

If you can eliminate stress you can eliminate cortisol from being released. Getting a sufficient amount of vitamin C in your diet can also correct cortisol levels.

Having less cortisol in your system not only means a lower accumulation of newly stored fat, it also lets your body know that you don't need the stored fat that you already have. This equals **weight loss**!

Because vitamin C is a soluble vitamin that gets eliminated in your urine it's important to eat sufficient amount of vitamin C daily in order to lose body fat. The high consumption of fruits and vegetables on the DASH diet enables you to keep your vitamin C intake high.

Tips to maximize your weight loss

Choose low-calorie foods

You can lose weight on the DASH diet by eating foods that have fewer calories. The key to losing weight is to burn more calories than you eat in a day.

Exchange sweets and other high calorie foods for low calorie foods like fruits and vegetables. Eat smarter, eat smaller portions, eat slowly and be a smart shopper.

Low-fat frozen yogurt will save you nearly 70 calories when compared to full-fat ice cream. Buy low-fat or fat-free when it is available and cut back on portion size.

If you want a snack, choose fresh fruit rather than a cookie or candy. This will increase your fruit consumption and save you about 80 calories per snack.

Dried fruits are a better choice than chips or pork rinds and will save you about 230 calories per snack.

If you have to buy canned fruit make sure it is packaged in water and not syrup.

Plan ahead

Buy an assortment of vegetables, slice them and take them to work along with a sandwich. This will increase your vegetable consumption and it will help you resist the temptation to grab a bag of chips from the vending machine at lunch. Replacing a bag of chips with vegetables will save you about 120 calories.

Choose healthy snacks

Eat healthy snacks without adding unhealthy seasonings. Try popcorn cooked in olive oil and seasoned with garlic or grated parmesan cheese rather than butter and salt.

Choose water

Drink water with a twist of lemon or lime rather than sodas and sweetened teas.

Adhere to recommended serving sizes

Watch your serving sizes on labels.

Consume less sodium

Sodium will make you retain water and it will cause inflammatory responses throughout your body. You need some sodium but not a lot.

Set a goal to watch your sodium intake and start paying attention to the information on food labels.

Prepackaged foods can contain excessive amounts of sodium.

Aim to buy foods that do not have salt added to them.

Note: Watch the salt content in canned foods, sauces, tomato juices and prepared foods.

Be creative and exchange salt with exotic spices when cooking meals. Let salt be your last resort.

Go low-fat

Choose lower fat methods of preparing your food such as baking, broiling and grilling.

Also, reduce the amount of oil and margarine that you use when cooking and use low-fat condiments.

Be smart about eating out

For eating out, do some research on the restaurant that you are going to by looking them up online to see how they prepare their food? You can get their menu online and find out how they cook their food.

Look for low sodium foods, low-fat, low calorie and special areas on the menu that offer lighter meal plans. If you do not see them ask your server.

Nutribullet Diet

Nutribullet is a widely popular superfood extractor that can help you achieve your health and fitness goals. The patented technology in Nutribullet will enable you to prepare high quality smoothies, soups, and many other healthy meals easily.

Each drink and dish in this recipe book is guaranteed to come out smooth and creamy yet retain the pulp for fiber content, as long as you use the Nutribullet correctly. Choose from a variety of energy smoothies that you can drink first thing in the morning, green smoothies to help you get your daily amount of vegetables, detox smoothies to help cleanse and revitalize your digestive system, and soups that will keep you satiated and well-nourished. Bring out the full potential of your Nutribullet and maximize its amazing features. You will soon discover how easy it actually is to prepare tasty and healthy drinks and dishes within the comforts of your own home.

Thanks again for downloading this book, I hope you enjoy it!

The Nutribullet in your Kitchen

It seems that everyone nowadays lives such busy lives that they tend to turn to quick and easy meal solutions in order to stay sane. Well, this may be the reason why smoothies are immensely popular among urban households. Smoothies take only a few minutes to prepare and are much healthier compared to microwave meals and fast food.

However, what a lot of people do not know is that the blender plays a crucial role in properly extracting nutrients from the ingredients. Cheap and low quality blenders tend to expose the delicate fruits, vegetables, and other ingredients to a certain level of heat that it ends up destroying most of the nutrients. You then end up consuming a much lower amount of nutrients than what you bargained for.

It is important to invest instead in a blender that will not only make it easy for you to process your smoothies but also contribute to retaining the best nutritional value from your chosen ingredients. The Nutribullet is one such blender that is reputed to have helped thousands of people from all over the world make smoothies that have helped them lose weight, gain energy, and improve their overall health.

How the Nutribullet Works

The Nutribullet, which is marketed as "The Superfood Extractor" is designed to do just that: it breaks down the ingredients by pulverizing it all to make the smoothest possible smoothie. This extraction process will make it easier for your body to absorb the nutrients from the ingredients and quickly distribute it throughout your cells.

The Nutribullet works on a powerful 600-watt motor and with what is called the "Extractor" blades (which are actually patented, by the way) that are sharp enough to completely break down even the hardest of root vegetables, nuts, stems, and seeds. The motor applies a so called "cyclonic action" that easily pulverizes the ingredients, including ice, without you having to shake or poke at the mixture every now and then.

Nutribullet has three types of blades that you can choose from depending on your needs. For instance, crushing ice and turning nuts, seeds, and grains into flour require different blades compared to the one that you will use for smoothies alone.

One major advantage of owning a Nutribullet is that it is so compact to the point of being portable. It can be stored quite easily because of its shape and size, despite the fact that you can blend up to 24 ounces of ingredients. Also, apart from smoothies, it can be used to mill nuts, grains, and seeds into meal, flour, and butter.

Another thing to be happy about the Nutribullet is that its cups are BPA-free, which means that the cups do not contain the toxic chemical called phthalates. However, since the cups still contain plastic, you must remember to never pour anything hot or even warm inside the cups. For hot soup recipes, let the soup cool down to room temperature completely first before pouring it into the Nutribullet cup, then heat up the soup again after blending.

The Proper Way to Use your Nutribullet

There are three pieces which constitute the Nutribullet: the first is the base which holds the processor engine, the second piece is the tops that contain the blade attachment, and the last is a "bullet" shaped (conical and oval) glass cup.

To use the Nutribullet safely and effectively, you start by placing the ingredients into the cup, attach the blade attachment on top not unlike a lid to a jar, and then start blending. Take note that you should never go beyond the "MAX" line of the cup when you are filling it up with ingredients. Going beyond this line will cause the ingredients to overflow and cause a mess that you will have to spend more time cleaning up than preparing your smoothies.

To transfer the smoothie from the blender, simply remove the cup from the processor, turn it upside down, detach the blade attachment, and pour the smoothie from the cup to your glass.

Once you have finished using your Nutribullet, you can easily clean it by following any one of the two tips. The first method is to detach the blade attachment and cup and rinse them in a basin of water, and then place them in the dishwasher. The second is by pouring soapy water into the cup and connecting it back to the blade attachment. Run the blender very quickly, then rinse and set aside to dry. Make sure that any residue is rinsed off thoroughly; otherwise, any trapped bits of ingredients will contaminate your next smoothie.

Fast Metabolism Diet

If you have ever tried dieting before, you know how difficult it can be to manage to keep the weight off once it has fallen off. People find it very difficult to diet because they are constantly trying to limit their portions, avoid eating sweets, and overall trying too hard. When it comes to dieting, you need to focus on a lifestyle change and not on "dieting". When people think they cannot have something, they will tend to want it more and this is why many diet programs just do not work.

The goal of dieting is not to just lose weight but to also lose body fat as well. What is the point of just losing weight but keeping all that fat packed on? One of the best ways to burn your fat is to make sure you are always eating the right amount of carbohydrates, protein, and fat. These three nutrients are needed for your body and you must make sure to take in enough of them before you can begin to boost your metabolism and see the fat and weight shed right off.

In addition to eating correctly, you will want to make sure that you are exercising and providing your body with the workout that it needs. Working out will help to strengthen your muscles and also build them as you start eating differently. You will begin to see results and notice that your fat is melting away and turning into pure muscle.

It is important to make sure that you are always providing yourself with a busy activity to do. Resting and not staying on the go will only cause your metabolism to stabilize and you can pack on the pounds again. You do not have to constantly be running or exercising but it is important to make sure you are walking around or doing something to keep your body moving.

One way to make sure that you are staying on track with your diet is to keep a journal of what you are eating every day. It can be easy to forget what you ate two days ago or how much protein was in your dinner last night. If you keep a record of this, you will be able to see what you are doing and always monitor your progression.

One way to be successful when you are working on transforming your body is to make sure that you are not sticking to just one thing. This means change up your diet and also change up your exercise routine. Constantly doing the same thing will become boring and will make you want to quit and give up. If you are trying new foods and cooking different dinners throughout the week, you will not become bored and tired of the food you are eating. Changing your workout routine will also allow you to enjoy new activities.

Clean-Eating Diet

What is Clean Eating?

Contrary to what most people believe, this practice is not a diet. But rather, clean eating is a lifestyle. This is not something that you can follow just to lose weight and forego once you have achieved your weight loss goals. Eating clean is a practice that you and your family should ultimately live by for the rest of your lives.

The concept of clean eating has been practiced ever since the first man learned how to make use of the natural vegetation and wild animal resources in their areas. It is simply eating organic, lean and naturally obtained fruits, vegetables and meat using the simplest and the healthiest preparations.

To better understand what this healthy lifestyle is all about, you definitely need to find out more about its principles.

This is because you need to do some major changes in your life especially if you have been leading an unhealthy lifestyle by eating mostly junk foods, processed foods, or instant meals. Clean eating is not the same as those diet fads that promise to help you lose weight. This is more about improving the quality of food that you eat than limiting the quantity. It also has something to do with changing your eating habits and your lifestyle.

Most of the food items included in the clean eating diet plan are also recommended by public health groups and organizations. Compared to diet fads, clean eating is more flexible and can be adapted to almost all kinds of lifestyle.

To help you understand what clean eating is, you need to know the basic principles of clean eating. Check out the paragraphs below.

Principles of clean eating

Whole Foods is the Best

Whole foods are foods that have not been processed and are in their most natural state. For example, whole grains are grains that still contain all the original layers or parts including the endosperm, germ, and bran. Grains that are crushed, cracked, or rolled are already considered processed. Natural foods are those that do not have any chemicals or artificial ingredients in them. Whole natural foods contain all the nutrients that are found in the original nutritional value of the food.

Unrefined vs Refined Foods

Refined foods are processed foods that no longer have all the nutrients that they originally had. Certain foods have to undergo this process to improve their taste, give them a longer shelf life, and create a finer appearance and texture. One example is refined white sugar. It is best to choose unrefined brown sugar than white sugar for your coffee or tea. However, when it comes to baking, most recipes require the use of white sugar because it gives a smoother and silkier texture to the bread or pastry. But if you want to get the complete nutrients of the food, you have to make sure that you choose unrefined over refined food products

Gives You the Cooking Independence

Meals prepared at home are known and proven to be several times healthier than your favorite fast food meals. No matter how much these restaurants claim that they use nothing but the best products, you can never be too sure that they do not use processed food products. Clean eating will help you learn how to prepare fast, simple and healthy meals.

Consume more Fruits and Vegetables

One thing that all diet plans and diet fads have in common is that all of them promote eating more fruits and vegetables. Everyone knows how beneficial fruits and vegetables are to your health. They contain vitamins and minerals that your body needs without having to worry about adding more calories. Fruits and vegetables also make you feel full longer, which prevents you from overeating. When choosing fruits and vegetables, be sure to pick those that came directly from the farm. You can buy fresh fruits and vegetables from your local farmer's market or stalls that sell produce.

Consume less saturated fats.

Fats in general are not bad to your health, contrary to popular belief. However, there is a specific kind of fats that you need to avoid called saturated fats. These fats are found in dairy products and meat. Clean eating does not mean that you should completely eliminate fats from your diet; in fact, that is not recommended because fats are also important to your health. What you need is to focus on good fats such as those found in canola oil, olive oil, nuts, and fish.

Lesser sodium Intake.

The daily recommendation for sodium is only 2300 mg per day and most Americans eat 1,000 mg more sodium than the limit because they often eat fast foods and processed foods. To ensure that your sodium intake is still within the limit, you should consider eating out less frequently and cooking your own food at home. You can make your meals tastier even without adding too much salt by using spices and herbs.

Reduce Meat Consumption.

Meat has saturated fats that are bad for your health. However, you cannot completely eliminate meat from your diet because it is an important source of protein. What you can do is to use meat as flavoring to your meals instead of serving it as the meal itself. For example, instead of eating fried chicken for dinner, you should consider adding bits of chicken in your soup.

No to high calorie drinks.

Instead of drinking soft drinks or specialty coffees that are high in calories, you should consider drinking plain water instead. In the morning, you can drink low-fat skim milk, unsweetened tea, or freshly squeezed fruit juice for breakfast.

Eat 5 to 6 small meals in a day.

The clean eating diet plan encourages people to eat small meals about five to six times a day instead of eating two or three large meals. Skipping meals is not encouraged and eating healthy snacks in between meals is encouraged. This prevents you from overeating and keeps your energy level stable throughout the day.

Reduce your alcohol intake.

You can still drink alcohol but you should limit your alcohol intake and avoid getting drunk. For women, the recommended limit for alcohol is one drink per day. For men, the limit is 2 drinks per day. Too much alcohol is bad for your health because it can cause dehydration and can add calories to your diet.

No to Processed Foods

Canned, packed and labeled foods are considered to be processed types of food. The thing about such types of foods is that they may contain ingredients, such as preservatives that could be chemically laced and are harmful to your body. But if there are processed foods that you can eat, those would be whole grain pastas, vegan meat substitutes, organic grains and flours and cheeses. Every time you read the labels, keep in mind that if you cannot pronounce it, do not buy it!

Lessen your sugar intake.

Aside from sodium, you should also watch your sugar intake. The recommended sugar intake is 9 teaspoons for men and 6 teaspoons for women. You should avoid sugary foods like baked treats, candies, and soda. You should also watch out for healthy foods with added sugar like cereal, yogurt, and tomato sauce.

Right Combination of Carbs and Protein is the Key

This will encourage you to go for more balanced meals every single day. Whether you are snacking or having lunch, your plate should have the right proportions of carbs and protein. This will not only make your healthier, you will also be able to quell all your bouts of hunger and unrealistic cravings.

Benefits of Clean Eating

Because of the kinds of food that you are encouraged to eat with the clean eating diet plan, you can get a lot of benefits that help improve your health. Some of the benefits of eating clean are listed in the paragraphs below.

Energy Booster

Getting the right kind and amount of nutrients helps boost your energy. For example, iron and vitamin B-complex improves cellular functions. Clean eating also promotes eating small meals more frequently. This helps regulate the sugar level in your blood stream which gives you a steady supply of energy throughout the day. This is also due to your reduced consumption of sweets and refined carbohydrates.

Improves your digestive system's processes

Have you noticed that after eating that large serving of cheese burger and a handful of fries, your stomach feels so full and totally acidic? Well, if you observe carefully, you will even hear your digestive enzymes struggle to work their way through all the oily processed foods that you have consumed. Clean eating will help put a stop to acid refluxes, indigestion and poor bowel movement. You will have all the fiber that you need to improve your digestion in so many ways.

Lose Weight Effectively

The kinds of food that you eat if you practice clean eating also help you lose weight. For instance, it promotes low sugar intake that helps you achieve optimum weight. It also encourages you to eat more fruits and vegetables and less meat which lowers your calorie intake. Aside from eating healthy foods, clean eating also promotes an active lifestyle. You can do some exercises or being more physically active can help you lose weight.

Lessen the feeling of Hunger

Junk food makes you crave more food, which in turn makes you gain those unwanted pounds. Eating cleaner and healthier food will make sure that you will feel full and satisfied longer since you will be completely nourished.

Boost Immunity

Eating clean foods also protects you against diseases like heart diseases, stroke, diabetes, and cancer. It helps lower your cholesterol level and boosts the strength of your blood vessels. Fruits and vegetables are also rich in vitamins and minerals that promote strong immunity that helps you fight illnesses. And because you are eating less saturated fat, the cholesterol level in your body is also regulated. The artificial and chemical ingredients in processed foods also increase risk of cancer. Fruits and vegetables are rich in antioxidants and phytonutrients that are known to help fight cancer cells.

Cooking is more fun

This lifestyle does not mean that you have to eat bland and dull looking meals every single time. Clean eating, with all the amazingly healthy ingredients that you can choose from, should and will encourage you to try new recipes to bring life to your dishes. Clean eating should get you excited to prepare your own meals!

Mental Health Improver

Aside from improving your physical health, eating clean foods also helps boost your mental health. Fish is rich in omega-3 fatty acids, a good kind of fat included in the clean eating diet plan. This fat helps fight depression and moodiness. Vitamin B-6, which can be found in sunflower seeds, pistachio nuts, and tuna, also helps produce dopamine, a hormone in the body that makes you feel good and happy.

Good for Everyone

Gone are the days when you think that healthy or clean eating is just for vegans, vegetarians, diabetes, heart patients or those who are on a really strict diet. Clean eating is for those who would like to take great care of themselves better.

Skin Enhancer

If you are healthy from within, your outward appearance will also look healthy which includes your hair and skin. Some fruits and vegetables are rich in antioxidants that are known to fight wrinkles and skin blemishes. Fruits and vegetables also have higher water content, which keeps your skin hydrated at all times. You also do not have to worry about chemicals that can be harmful to your body and can cause damage to your skin.

Clean Eating Tips That Will You Lose Weight Effectively

It is important that you know some useful tips that will help you lose weight and rejuvenate. You also need to know some tips on how to make clean and green eating a permanent part of your life. Remember that this is not just a diet fad that you only need to do for a limited timeframe. This requires significant changes in your routine and your life in general, which is why it is important that you plan the transition carefully. Here are some tips and ideas you might find useful.

Get plenty of exercise

Changing your diet alone is not enough to achieve your optimum weight and health. You also need to get the right amount of exercise that your body needs to burn the calories you get from the food you eat and prevent them from turning into fat. You need to exercise regularly if you want to lose weight and to keep yourself healthy. You can do some cardio workout and muscle and strength training that will help you lose weight and become more fit and healthy. You can either pay for a monthly gym membership where you have a personal trainer, or do the exercises yourself at the park or at home.

Aside from regular workouts, you can also get enough exercise by being more physically active. Instead of driving your car to buy a carton of milk at the grocery just a couple of blocks away from your house, you should consider walking or riding your bike. Instead of using the elevator, you can use the stairs to go to your office floor, unless of course your office is located on the 23rd floor or something. If that's the case, you should consider riding the elevator halfway or two-thirds up then using the stairs for the remaining few floors.

Spice Up Your Meals

If you are a bit scared to try new spices and seasoning blends, why don't you go for herbs and other ingredients that could elevate and take your healthy meals to whole new levels? Try experimenting and incorporating these healthy herbs and spices in your next recipes:

- Cloves
- Cinnamon
- Nutmeg
- Cumin
- Turmeric
- Sage
- Mint
- Rosemary
- Basil
- Marjoram
- Chili
- Thyme

Get enough sleep and rest

Getting enough sleep and rest is also a part of a clean lifestyle. Resting or sleeping makes your body refreshed and rejuvenated the next day. This will allow you to perform your tasks more efficiently. It is also easier to follow your clean eating lifestyle if you have enough energy. For example, you will have the energy to prepare clean meals throughout the day and do some exercises if your body is well-rested.

Plan your meals

There are several ways to diversify your meals on a daily basis. Make the internet your best friend to look for amazingly delicious but unbelievably healthy dishes that you can easily make for your family. You can create a chart and plan what you will be cooking and eating for a week or in the next few days.

Learn the different recommendations for food groups

Clean eating is also about balanced eating. Eating whole, natural foods will be useless if you do not get the recommended amount of all the food groups. You need to know what foods are great sources of protein, carbohydrates, good fats, vitamins, minerals, fiber, and other nutrients that your body needs. It is important to get the recommended amount of each of these nutrients in your diet because they have different functions that keep you healthy and improve your general well-being. For instance, fiber's main function is to flush out toxins in your body and improve your bowel movement. Protein, on the other hand, improves your strength and muscles.

Vegan Diet

Veganism and Its Benefits

There are many reasons why people choose the vegan lifestyle. It is certainly better to eat plant based foods than the usual American diet which contains a lot of fat and sugar in different forms. We feed on fast-food and we drink gallons of fizzy drinks. How can that be beneficial for our body and mind?

Being healthy and energetic can only be done with healthy and nutritious food. For that reason, veganism is not a diet, but a lifestyle and philosophy. Being vegan means that you eat only plant based foods. Nothing organic should be included in your diet nor in every other aspects of your life, such as cosmetics or clothing.

Let's look more deeply into the benefits of the vegan lifestyle so we can get a clear picture of it. The first thing you should be concerned about is fat. Our common diet is loaded with fat, even products that you wouldn't suspect. Dr. Michael Klaper, one of the promoters of veganism, in one of his famous presentations called *Food That Kills*, warns us that fat is the main cause of death nowadays. He goes on saying that without knowing it, we eat pure fat found everywhere, from yogurt to chocolate and of course, butter and meat.

What he basically says is that our body and digestive system is not ready to eat various fat loaded foods. For instance, dairy products. Milk is designed to feed calves, not people. Its chemical compounds aren't designed to be digested by our system, but for cows and their babies. The milk itself is loaded with fats and protein that help the calves grow.

However, people take milk, skim its fat and turn it into products like yogurt, sour cream, cheese, chocolate or whipping cream. Since your system is not ready for such a large amount of fat, it tries to deal with it as best as possible and often it deposits it in places you wouldn't even think about, such as arteries and your heart, liver or pancreas.

The other downside of this is that this kind of products, a mix of dairy and sugars usually, can develop addictions we're not aware of. You may often crave for sweet or milk products and eating those makes you feel better. That is why a chocolate bar is able to elevate your mood in such a good way.

The food industry went from no fat to low fat in the last few years and that is because people start to realize how important fat can be. However, there is a difference between the fat that is good for your body and the fat that causes more harm than anything else. There are fats who, surprisingly, lower cholesterol and the risk of heart disease and those are the fats found in avocado, sunflower oil, olive oil or walnuts. But then there are saturated fats, found in meat and dairy products who increase cholesterol and also the risks of blood clots and heart attacks.

At the same time, fruits and vegetables have no fat and are loaded with vitamins, nutrients and their content makes them very easy to digest and absorb. Fibers are one of the best things we get from fresh fruits and veggies. They promote a healthy digestive system which then leads to an improved immune system. Let's not forget about antioxidants as well as they are the ones who flush out all the toxins from your body, boosting its ability to fight against viruses or bacteria even more.

In the end, a diet consisting of more fruits and vegetables can only benefit us and the great thing is that it will show on the outside as well. Don't you want a healthy looking skin? Don't you want to get that glow in your eyes back? You will shine and glow in a way that it will not stay unnoticed.

Checklist No. 4

1. Do you prefer Paleo Diet?

A. Yes

B. Somewhat

C. Unsure

D. Not at all

2. Do you think Dash Diet is applicable to you?

A. Yes

B. Somewhat

C. Unsure

D. Not at all

3. Is fast metabolism diet effective in losing weight on women?

A. Yes

B. Somewhat

C. Unsure

D. Not at all

4. According to what you have read, is Nutribullet Diet applicable to all especially to women?

A. Yes

B. Somewhat

C. Unsure

D. Not at all

5. Do you think Clean Eating Diet is the most recommended diet lifestyle for women?

A. Yes

B. Somewhat

C. Unsure

D. Not at all

6. Is vegan diet applicable to you?

A. Yes

B. Somewhat

C. Unsure

D. Not at all

7. Would you try any of these suggested diets in these chapter?

A. Yes

B. Somewhat

C. Unsure

D. Not at all

Chapter 5:

Secret of Transformation

Cycle 1: Accelerate

The very first thing you should understand in losing weight especially in women is cleansing your body of any sugar craving by means of sugar detoxification. This not only promotes healthy digestion but also accelerates the process of fat burning in your body.

There are different types of sugars; glucose (a natural sugar found in fruits), sucrose (sugar you buy at the store), and fructose (the only sugar that humans don't naturally produce themselves.)

When consuming large amounts of sugar, the body uses the liver to metabolize most of the fructose. The fructose is then turned into fat and stows it away into the blood. Your glucose levels rise when you consume meals that have a lot of carbs. However, too much glucose is toxic and your insulin level rises as well to get rid of the glucose into the cells and out of the bloodstream. Without the proper function of your insulin, the blood glucose levels would extent to deadly levels. Although insulin saves your life on a regular basis, the effect it has basically turns energy from the food into fat cells.

Why Detox?

As previously stated, there are different types of sugars; however some have more negative effects than others. There are three types of carbohydrates that are in foods: starch, sugar, and fiber. The capacity of sugar molecules in certain sugars range; simple sugars like fructose, lactose, and sucrose only have one or two molecules, while fiber and starch are complex carbohydrates that can contain hundreds of sugar molecules. Due to their large amounts of sugar molecules, complex carbohydrates enter the bloodstream slowly and take longer to digest. Although simple sugars quickly enter the bloodstream, they cause the blood sugar to spike. Any "bad" sugar that you consume is simple sugar; however not all simple sugars are bad. What matters is the source in which your body receives the sugar, which is why keeping to a low sugar diet is important, especially for weight loss.

A detox resets your metabolism so that it burns carbohydrates and fat in a more functional and natural way, helping to burn fat. Although the end goal is to stick to the diet to the point that it becomes a lifestyle.

Why removing sugar from diet is difficult

Sugar is a highly addictive compound. Over the years, the human body has developed a proclivity for sweet foods as a survival mechanism since sugar is one of the easiest and the quickest source of energy. As with any other forms of dependence from toxic substances (e.g. alcohol, nicotine from cigarettes, etc.,), withdrawal is a very traumatic experience—both emotionally and physiologically. This is because the pleasure pathway created by sugar consumption over extended periods of time always becomes strongly reinforced.

Eliminating sugar from the diet

There are two ways to give a solution to sugar addiction and to remove sugar from the body while minimizing or altogether eliminating the negative effects of withdrawal: gradually reducing the sugar consumption over time or replacing sugar with a substance that gives the same quality and level of pleasure when consumed. The pleasure derived from sugar consumption stems from its sweetness. As a survival response learned through evolution, the body has acquired the tendency to associate sweetness with pleasure. Apart from saltiness, no other taste elicits the same neural response.

The second method of eliminating sugar from the body requires the consumption of a substance the gives the impression of sweetness minus the sugar. A number of substances developed and discovered over the years give this result. These substances are referred to as sweeteners owing to their ability to activate the sweet receptors in the tongue without sugar.

Cycle 2: Activate

You may be tempted to cut as many calories as you can in your diet. A large deficit should lead to more pounds lost. Right? Wrong!

By severely lowering a number of calories in your diet, your body will reduce the metabolic rate. So it will get into survival mode thereby conserving fat instead of burning. This will not lead to more weight lost, but you will only starve yourself.

The best way is to regulate your calorie intake by means of gradual increasing and decreasing your calorie intake so it can stimulate fat burning in your body thus resetting your body metabolism. This makes the body metabolize more fat thus resulting to weight loss.

Cycle 3: Achieve

Changing your eating habits does not happen overnight. It must align with your goal to a more healthy living. Thus gradual changes are necessary and additional introduction of other foods must be done in a gradual manner. Here are some tips in achieving your goal towards losing weight.

Change gradually

If you currently only eat one or two servings of fruits and vegetables a day try adding a serving at lunch and one at dinner.

Rather than switching to an "all or nothing" approach to whole grains, start by making one or two of your grain serving's whole grains.

Increasing fruits, vegetables and whole grains gradually can help prevent bloating or diarrhea that may occur if you aren't used to eating high-fiber diet.

Reward successes and forgive slip-ups

Reward yourself with a nonfood treat for your accomplishments such as renting a movie, purchasing a book or getting together with a friend.

Everyone slips up sometimes especially when learning something new. Remember that changing your lifestyle is a long-term process. Find out what triggered your setback then pick up where you left off.

Make exercise an important part of your diet lifestyle

Any diet plan will improve your health and make you lose weight all on its own. However, if you make regular exercise a habit you will boost your body's ability to shed unwanted pounds.

When you combine diet with a good amount of physical activity (30 minutes/day of moderate exercise) it will also maximize your ability to reduce blood pressure.

Get support if you need it

If you are having trouble sticking to the diet talk to your doctor or dietitian about it. They may be able to offer some tips that will help you stick to the diet more effectively.

Cycle 4: Arrive

The most important part for every diet plan to be successful is that you enjoy what you are doing. Many of women are willing to undertake any diet plan but in return they live miserable lives.

Rewarding yourself once in a while is the perfect reinforcement to make your diet plan more fun and enjoyable. Depriving yourself so much is not a good idea. It only makes your cravings uncontrollable. Eating what you really like once in a while in moderation is always a good diet plan than suffering from severe deprivation which only creates more possibilities of relapses.

Checklist No. 5

1. Are you aware that too much intake of sugar in your body can have a bad effects on your health?

A. Yes

B. Somewhat

C. Unsure

D. Not at all

2. Do you feel you have a sugar addiction?

A. Yes

B. Somewhat

C. Unsure

D. Not at all

3. Is achieving the ideal weight important to you?

A. Yes

B. Somewhat

C. Unsure

D. Not at all

4. Do you feel you have some relapses in any of the said goals in transformation?

A. Yes

B. Somewhat

C. Unsure

D. Not at all

5. Are you willing to detoxify your body from any sweet cravings?

A. Yes

B. Somewhat

C. Unsure

D. Not at all

6. Do you feel that the said secrets are applicable to you?

A. Yes

B. Somewhat

C. Unsure

D. Not at all

7. Can you agree that you can achieve the goals said in this chapter?

A. Yes

B. Somewhat

C. Unsure

D. Not at all

Chapter 7:

Cleansing and Detoxification

Cleanse diet has become a very popular way to get healthy and lose excess weight. It is important to know how to do the cleanse diet properly in order to feel good and stay healthy.

The cleanse diet is actually not a new thing. In the United States, cleanse diet became popular in the 1920s and 1930s. However, when the theories backing it lost support, it slowly fell out of favor. Currently, the idea of cleansing with the use of colon irrigation, enzymes or teas has experienced resurgence.

What is Cleanse?

The definition of cleanse is quite extensive. In its basic sense, cleanse is any type of lifestyle regimen or diet which is focused on detoxifying the body and bringing back optimum health. The sad part is, cleanse or cleansing is usually synonymous with eating disorders. However, cleansing can possibly be a vital part of a weight loss regimen if you use the right kind of cleanse or detox diet appropriate for your body and lifestyle.

What is the theory behind natural cleanse?

One of the primary theories behind cleanse or cleansing is a traditional belief referred to as the theory of autointoxication. The principle behind this belief is that the undigested food may lead to the buildup of mucus in the colon. This accumulation generates toxins, which poisons the body as it enters the bloodstream.

Most people reported that these toxins can lead to different symptoms, including the following:

- Low energy
- Weight gain
- Headache
- Fatigue

What is natural cleanse?

There are two primary methods of cleanse or cleansing: One involves seeing a health practitioner to have colon irrigation; and the other involves buying and using cleansing products.

1. Cleansing with colon irrigation (high colonics). Colonic hydro therapists or colonic hygienists conduct colon irrigations. Colon irrigations work like an enema, although they involve no discomfort and odors and much more water. During colon irrigation, you lie on a table, and then a gravity-based reservoir or a low-pressure pump flushes several gallons of water through a tiny tube that's inserted into the rectum.

A therapist may massage the abdomen after the water is in the colon. The water is then released like a regular bowel movement. This procedure flushes out the wastes and fluids. The whole process may be repeated. A session may usually last up to an hour.

The health care provider may use various temperatures and water pressures. The use of probiotics, coffee, herbs and enzymes may also be employed.

2. Cleansing with the use of liquid or powdered supplements. This involves taking some supplements for cleansing by mouth or taken through the rectum. Either way, the principle behind this is to help the colon get rid of its contents. These cleansing products may be bought in supermarkets, pharmacies or health food stores. They include:

- Magnesium

- Enzymes

- Herbal teas

- Laxatives – both stimulant and non-stimulant kinds

- Enemas

What is the Goal of Cleansing?

Colon irrigation practitioners and producers of colon cleansing products claim broad and wide-reaching health benefits of cleansing. Their ultimate objective is to clean up the colon from huge amounts of stagnant, potentially toxic waste accumulated on the colon walls. Doing a cleanse, as they claim, will improve the natural vigor of the body.

Other stated goals of doing a cleanse include the following:

- Lessening the risk of developing colon cancer

- Weight loss

- Boosting the immune system

- Improving mental outlook

Cleansing has been the subject of studies in relation to a number of health issues, including the following:

- Before and during bowel surgeries

- Drug withdrawal

- Spasm during colonoscopy

- Ostomy or the surgical relation between the outside of the body and the intestine

- Fecal incontinence

The Benefits of a Cleanse Diet

Cleansing diets can help in improving the body's general health and wellness. It can even reduce the risks of developing colon cancer. Below is a list of some of the claimed benefits of a cleanse diet:

1. Enhances the body's well-being. Cleansing the colon from toxins and wastes may be achieved by releasing layers of colon buildup. This can bring about feelings of strength and lightness, as well as overall good health and wellbeing.

2. Maintains proper pH balance in the bloodstream. Foods that lead to colon blockages produce acids, specifically a diet abundant in protein without sufficient fiber. This results to overall malaise in the body. The tissues in the colon eventually become inflamed and damaged, weakening the colon. The colon may not be effective in its function of allowing only vitamins, minerals and water to pass into the bloodstream. If fecal matter, parasites, fungus, molds and yeasts enter the bloodstream and connected tissue, the pH level of the body will be thrown out of balance.

3. Enhances fertility. Cleanse diet involves the intake of increased amounts of fiber and health food choices. It also keeps weight under control. Fat is based on estrogen. If too much fat is present, the chance of becoming pregnant is relatively low. A colon which is weighed down by years of accumulation can also adversely affect the uterus, as well as the surrounding reproductive organs in females, causing strain.

Cleansing diet helps in ridding the body of many toxins and harmful chemicals that adversely affect the sperm and egg. A lot of natural health practitioners suggest that both partners try cleansing diets before attempting pregnancy.

4. Lessens the risk of developing colon cancer. All the toxic substances that you breathe in, drink, eat and absorb through the skin are broken down by the liver and gastrointestinal system. If these harmful substances are not eliminated from the liver and colon as fast as possible, they can damage the body's systems. By getting rid of stagnant body waste, you lessen the causes and risk of developing cancerous growths, cysts and polyps in the colon and the gastrointestinal tract.

5. Kick-starts weight loss. Food items, which are low in fiber, transport through the digestive tract at a much slower pace than those that are abundant in fiber. These slow-moving food items generate excess mucous that tend to stick to the walls of the intestine. This will eventually drag down the intestinal tract with excess pounds of decaying fecal materials.

Cleansing diet also helps in weight reduction. Many people have claimed to lose weight up to 20 pounds over only a month. A cleansing diet can lead to dramatic weight loss and jump-start your metabolism. It can also lead your interests to better food choices and overall wellness.

6. Enhances concentration. Ineffective vitamin absorption as well as poor diet can make you more distracted and lose concentration. The accumulation of mucous and toxic substances in the colon can prevent the body from obtaining what it needs to function optimally. Cleaning up the colon with a cleansing diet can be the key to better concentration and alertness. Its effects can greatly affect your overall health, and also your work and relationships.

7. Boosts the body's ability to effectively absorb vitamins and nutrients. A clean colon works effectively in allowing only vitamins, nutrients and water to be absorbed into the bloodstream, rather than releasing bacteria and toxic material through the walls of the colon. When the colon is cleansed, it clears up the way for important vitamins and nutrients to filter into the body unhampered

8. Enhances the digestive system's effectiveness. As the colon is cleansed, it eliminates undigested wastes out of the body, clearing the way for the good nutrients to be absorbed effectively. If the toxic materials and wastes stay in the body for a long time, it becomes a breeding ground for illnesses and bad bacteria. A clean colon through a cleansing diet allows toxic materials from undigested waste to pass easily through the digestive tract.

9. Maintains the regularity of bowel movements and prevents constipation. Constipation, particularly when it is chronic, leads to sluggish digestive response. This will make the wastes stay longer in the digestive system. This condition will increase the chances of toxic materials released into the bloodstream. This will become the cause of irritations and other health problems such as varicose veins and hemorrhoids.

Foods to Avoid

You would be shocked to learn that a good percentage of the food you eat, under the impression that it is healthy, can make you gain weight. You may think that just a bit of it now and then will not do much harm. But it is only when you see yourself gaining weight that you realize how dangerous such food is.

Breakfast Cereals –

Starting the day with the right food is crucial as it determines your productivity throughout the day. And for many people, cereals are the definition of the right breakfast. These foods, unfortunately, are packed with a lot of sugar. So in the end, insulin levels rise thereby stopping the burning of fat.

Low-Fat Yogurt –

Yogurt is certainly one of the healthiest foods in the world, but mostly when you make it yourself. Store-bought yogurt is filled with unknown ingredients including sugar.

Fruit Juices –

Juices that are 100% fruit are not cheap. So to bring the cost down, most juices are fruit-flavored with a lot of sugar added to improve the taste. But even if the juice you drink is 100% fruit, the lack of fiber means you will still have a lot of sugar being absorbed into your blood stream, a situation that can lead to weight gain down the road.

Alcohol –

If you can't stop yourself from popping bottles every night, you now know what may be making your fat. As a solution, drink alcohol in moderation.

White Carbs –

Foods that have a high glycemic index are bound to make you fat if they are heavily present in your diet. Such food includes white rice, pasta, and white bread.

Gluten Free Food –

Gluten Free foods have become very popular recently. Unfortunately, they suffer from the same problem of having a lot of added sugar to improve taste. If you want gluten free food, make sure you choose food that is gluten free naturally.

Dried Fruits –

It's not all natural food that is good for you. Dried fruits, for example, are a no-no if you want to lose weight. They do not have a lot of fiber which means sugar is absorbed into your body at a faster rate.

Fried Foods –

Most foods are fried with unhealthy fats. So if you want to see the change you want, stay away from such food. Otherwise, you will add unnecessary calories into your diet which will ruin any chances of losing weight rapidly.

Processed Food –

If you depend on processed food, you do your body an injustice. Not only do you eat unknown ingredients, but you also ingest a lot of calories as such food is high in sugar, fats, and sodium.

Ideal Food for Cleansing

Food is really the best form of medicine when it comes to cleansing the body of harmful toxins. You will be amazed to find out that a lot of your favorite foods can cleanse the body's natural detoxification organs such as the skin, kidneys, intestines and liver. Cleansing will prevent harmful toxic accumulation. Help in ridding the adverse effects of second-hand smoke, food additives, pollution and other toxins by eating healthy and delicious foods such as the following:

- Cabbage – contains a number of antioxidant and anticancer substances that help the liver in breaking down excessive hormones. Cabbage can also cleanse the digestive tract and maintain some of the harmful substances found in cigarette fumes at bay. Cabbage can also boost the liver's natural ability to detoxify.

- Blueberries – is one of the most potent healing foods. Blueberries have natural aspirin that aids in reducing the tissue-damaging impacts of chronic inflammation, while reducing pain. It also serves as antibiotics by hampering bacterial entry in the urinary tract, thereby assisting in the prevention of infection. Blueberries also contain antiviral components which help in blocking toxins from crossing blood-brain barrier to obtain access to the delicate brain.

- Beets – contain a peculiar combination of natural plant substances which make them effective liver cleansers and blood purifiers.

- Avocados – are nutritional powerhouses that can dilate blood vessels and lessen cholesterol levels while blocking artery-damaging toxicity. Avocados contain a natural compound called glutathione, which blocks at least 30 various carcinogenic substances while helping the liver's natural ability to detoxify synthetic substances.

- Apples – are abundant in pectin, which is a kind of fiber that binds heavy metals and cholesterol in the body. Apples help largely in getting rid of toxin accumulation and cleansing the colon.

- Grapefruit – contains an abundant amount of pectin, which is a type of fiber that binds cholesterol molecules in the body, thereby cleansing the blood. Pectin fiber also binds heavy metals in the body as they are flushed out of the digestive system. Grapefruit also contains antiviral substances which help in cleansing dangerous viruses out of the body. Grapefruit is a potent liver and intestinal detoxifier.

- Garlic – helps in cleansing viruses, intestinal parasites and harmful bacteria from the body, particularly in the intestines and the blood. Garlic also aids in cleansing build up in the arteries and contain antioxidants and anti-cancer properties that help detoxify the body of dangerous substances. In addition to this, it helps with the cleansing of the respiratory tract by getting rid of mucus accumulation in the sinuses and the lungs. Choose only fresh garlic to take advantage of its numerous health benefits and not powdered garlic, which virtually does not contain any of the above-mentioned properties.

- Flaxseeds and flaxseed oil – contain abundant levels of essential fatty acids, specifically Omega 3. Flaxseed oil and flaxseed are important for a lot of cleansing activities all throughout the body.

- Celery and celery seed – are potent blood cleansers. They also contain a variety of anti-cancer substances that aid in detoxifying cancer cells out of the body. Celery and celery seeds have over twenty different anti-inflammatory compounds which are especially excellent for cleansing compounds found in cigarette fumes.

- Watercress – this delicious green may not be familiar for many but this can be an excellent choice for sandwiches since it can boost the activity of detoxification enzymes and acts on any present cancer cells throughout the body. According to current clinical studies, watercress can eliminate higher than average amounts of carcinogenic compounds among smokers, thereby eliminating them from the body.

Seaweed – while seaweed may have been the most underrated vegetable in western communities, according to scientific research, seaweeds bind to heavy metal waste in the body. Seaweed can also bind to radioactive wastes inside the body to help in flushing them out. Furthermore, seaweed is a powerhouse of trace minerals.

Lemons – contain huge amounts of Vitamin C, which makes them excellent liver detoxifiers. Vitamin C is required by the body to make an essential compound called glutathione, which aids the liver in detoxifying dangerous compounds in the body. To support your cleansing efforts regularly, add a squeeze of fresh lemon juice to pure water.

Legumes – are abundant with fiber that aids in reducing cholesterol levels, regulates blood sugar levels and cleanses the intestines. They also aid in safeguarding the body against all types of cancer.

Kale – contains potent antioxidant and anti-cancer properties that aid in cleansing the body of dangerous compounds. Kale is also abundant in fiber, which assists in cleansing the intestinal tract. Just like cabbage, kale aids in balancing out the compounds found in cigarette fumes and boosts the natural ability of the liver for cleansing.

Checklist No. 7

1. Do you feel that cleansing diet is necessary in losing weight especially in women?

A. Yes

B. Somewhat

C. Unsure

D. Not at all

2. Can you commit yourself to cleansing diet?

A. Yes

B. Somewhat

C. Unsure

D. Not at all

3. Do you feel that cleansing is not applicable to anyone?

A. Yes

B. Somewhat

C. Unsure

D. Not at all

4. Did you start already the cleansing diet? Do you feel any of the health benefits?

A. Yes

B. Somewhat

C. Unsure

D. Not at all

5. Are you aware that toxins in your body can be accumulated overtime due to unhealthy diet?

A. Yes

B. Somewhat

C. Unsure

D. Not at all

6. Do you know that an uncleansed body can hinder normal absorption of essential nutrients needed by your body?

A. Yes

B. Somewhat

C. Unsure

D. Not at all

7. If given any chance will you suggest cleansing diet to your friends?

A. Yes

B. Somewhat

C. Unsure

D. Not at all

Chapter 8:

NEAT (Non – Exercise Activity Thermogenesis)

What is NEAT (Non – Exercise Activity Thermogenesis)?

Non-Exercise Activity Thermogenesis (**N.E.A.T**) was created by Dr. James Levine who is credited for his extensive research on N.E.A.T. According to him, the calories that we intake can be expanded in two ways. One is the usual way and that is going to any local gym while the other one is doing all the daily activities which is called N.E.A.T (.Non-Exercise Activity Thermogenesis). It seems that N.E.A.T is far more effective in calorie burning than the usual exercise which often is not applicable to anyone.

In the dawn of the advance technology, most of the people have no time to go to the local gym to exercise and to burn calories. While most us are advocating the conventional way of high strung exercises which often needs considerable time, N.E.A.T offers a new and practical way of losing weight by understanding the proper distribution of calories in daily activities.

If the main goal of losing weight is burning the calories then N.E.A.T is far more practical and easier than going to a gym which oftentimes an ordinary busy person cannot afford to do so.

How NEAT helps to Lose Weight in Women

Proper information on the right amount of calorie intake in every activities is the key to the N.E.A.T lifestyle. Ordinary people are often ignorant on the right amount of calories they need every day. This results to unnecessary calories stored in our body producing unwanted fats.

If moving more is the key to loosening weight then the N.E.A.T lifestyle is the most natural way to burn calories. The right amount of calories intake versus the calories needed in the specific activity is the best way to lose weight properly.

Cardiovascular exercises are ideal for burning excessive fats and stress relieving but commitment is the only difference. Finding this high intensity exercise enjoyable will likely produce a more positive output than doing exercises which only cause more fatigue.

The N.E.A.T lifestyle offers more practical ways to burn calories resulting in a more natural way to lose weight. N.E.A.T teaches you to take any opportunity for physical activity in daily life. For example instead of taking the elevator, take the stairs. This is the best example of burning the calories in the natural way. Thus the N.E.A.T lifestyle is the best way to lose weight for people who have a busy lifestyle and no time to go to gym.

Checklist No. 8

1. Do you understand what N.E.A.T is all about?

A. Yes

B. Somewhat

C. Unsure

D. Not at all

2. Do you prefer conventional exercise over the N.E.A.T lifestyle?

A. Yes

B. Somewhat

C. Unsure

D. Not at all

3. Do you know what your daily ideal calorie intake is?

A. Yes

B. Somewhat

C. Unsure

D. Not at all

4. Do you think the N.E.A.T lifestyle is a more practical way to lose weight?

A. Yes

B. Somewhat

C. Unsure

D. Not at all

5. Are youthe type of person who love shortcuts in daily activities?

A. Yes

B. Somewhat

C. Unsure

D. Not at all

6. Do you think technology nowadays makes more people fatter?

A. Yes

B. Somewhat

C. Unsure

D. Not at all

7. Overall if you assess your lifestyle can you say that N.E.A.T is a more powerful way to lose weight than going to the local gym?

A. Yes

B. Somewhat

C. Unsure

D. Not at all

Chapter 9:

Effective Exercise Activities for Women

Exercise: The Cure for Fat

While trying to lose weight, you have probably come across a lot of different advice when it comes to exercise techniques. But the **best way to lose weight, hands down, is to strength train.** Strength training helps you build up lean muscles, which, in turn, enhances your metabolic rate. You will be able to burn fat 24/7 when you have plenty of lean muscle working for you.

Each extra pound of muscle needs about 40 to 50 calories to sustain itself. So if you can build about 20 pounds of muscles in your body, you will burn 800 to 1000 calories without having to do a thing. Once you work out, the effect continues for the next 48 hours, even when you are just relaxing or watching television.

Strength training is also important, not only because it helps add those attractive looking muscles, but also because it improves bone density, which is very important as we age.

Now, you might be wondering why I am asking you to strength train, because you do not want an abnormally muscular body. Do not worry. The abnormal muscles are truly abnormal, and you get them by use of steroids. And being a woman, there is no chance that you will ever develop those kind of muscles, because you have lower testosterone levels than men do.

You might also be wondering how long a muscle you have built stays. Muscles actually deteriorate with age, and that is one of the main reasons why even the fit people seem to gain weight overnight.

While you will find that muscle deterioration is out of your control, you can do what you can--continue to strength train so that the muscle that is deteriorating is replaced by a new set of lean muscles that burn your body fat effectively.

High Intensity Training

I will now give you an exercise schedule that you need to practice 3 times a week to get the body you have always wanted.

By high intensity, I mean exercising to the point at which your body cannot exercise anymore. For example, say that you can lift a weight of 50 lbs, ten times, but you have just lifted it 7 times. In this case, you have trained at only 70% intensity for the exercise and not 100%. We are aiming at 100% intensity exercises, or those that fully tire out your muscles.

When we do not work out until our maximum limit, the body does not feel the urge to develop more muscles or increase the strength of the muscle. Pushing it to the edge is a stimulus for the muscle to grow. It will grow because it has to prepare for the next high intensity workout.

Another thing about high intensity workouts is that the gap between exercise sets should be kept to a minimum. At most you should rest for only 30 seconds between sets. A gap of 2 to 3 minutes between sets, like they practice in most gyms, is not as effective.

How do you get the maximum benefit from high intensity exercise?

You have to increase it gradually and then reduce it gradually. Training more than what is necessary will only lead your muscles to wear out and get swollen, lacerated and infected.

What's the right volume and frequency?

If you strength train in the right volume and with the correct frequency, you will get stronger by the day, and that is how you know you have a frequency that is right for you.

If you are not feeling stronger, even after strength training, there is something that is going wrong with your training. You could either be exercising or too little (intensity), far too short or too long of a time (volume) or too often or not (frequency).

In fact, as you grow stronger, you should reduce the volume and frequency of training. This is because 50 pounds of muscles will get more fatigued and take more time to heal up than 25 pounds. So the ideal thing would be to reduce strength training, but not to stop it completely. If you give up or work out just once a month, it is not going to help. The muscles will again deteriorate and your metabolic rate will again fall, making you gain weight.

So it is true that only you can figure out how much of training is just right for you. But I, through this book, will help you figure out a perfect exercise plan for yourself, so that you get the body that you have been dreaming of.

What's double training?

As you strength train, you will build up new muscles and will have more strength. Your goal is to do 8 sets of 11 repetitions at a certain weight, so the next time you train, you should be able to do at least 12 repetitions or more of each exercise at that same weight. This is because the body acknowledges your failure and builds up more muscles and strength in them so that you are a little stronger when you practice it the next time.

When you can easily do more than 12 repetitions, increase the weight that you are lifting. So you will return back to your 8 sets and 11 repetitions, but you will soon be able to reach a higher number of sets and repeats. This is called **double training**. It is a very important aspect of strength training, as once your body gets used to something, it stops creating new muscles. So the idea is to have as many new muscles build as possible, so as to lose fat.

However, do not go overboard with your exercise plan. As you reach a certain level, you won't need to develop more muscles, only maintain what you have. After a certain point you have to reduce the strength training to some extent, but not stop it. Stopping it will again lead to the decay of muscles, therefore reducing metabolic rate and you will gain fat once again.

Once you start following the exercise pattern I have talked about, keeping these principles in mind and opting for a healthy lifestyle, you are sure to lose weight by gaining more muscles.

How many sets & repetition you should do?

High intensity exercise means you should repeat an exercise until you are not able to do even one repeat without rest.

On average, I recommend 2 to 3 seconds while lifting and 3 to 4 seconds while lowering. To get the best results and avoid the exercise turning into an endurance exercise, start off with a weight that is 70-80% of your limit for 1 repetition. You will find that you are able to repeat the exercise 8 to 10 times in a 40 to 70 second time period, following the 5-6 seconds per repeat I suggested.

How many sets to perform?

I believe one set performed well is more than sufficient, because you should have put 100% of effort into the 1st set. Doing it right and for a short while is the real secret to a healthy body and a peaceful mind.

I also recommend that you do full body workouts, as they balance the body better and takes less time. From my own experience, I can also tell you that cardiovascular fitness, strength training, and overall fitness are achieved better in the case of full body workouts.

I suggest a simple warm up, but make sure that the warm ups do not take up too much of your energy or become your main exercise.

Muscles are repaired and formed only after you stop exercising. Therefore, if you find that the workouts are not working on you, you perhaps are not giving the body enough time to repair itself. I suggest taking a day of rest between each workout day to begin with. As you start getting to know your body and your routine better, you can devise a schedule that works best for you.

While working out, always keep a water bottle handy and keep sipping cold water. You should never dehydrate your body while working out, as it will affect your workouts. Also keep a watch handy to keep track of time.

What's the correct breathing technique?

You should exhale while contracting your muscles and inhale while lengthening. While strength training, when you are pushing the weight away, your muscles contract and you should exhale, and while bringing them back in place your muscles relax and you should inhale.

But if you are doing the exercise as slowly as I suggest, you might require breathing more than once. There is nothing wrong in that. However, holding your breath during high intensity exercise can cause high blood pressure, hernia, dizziness, and all sorts of other ailments. So don't forget to breathe!

Determine Your Perfect Workout

Now that you are all equipped with the knowledge that is required for a perfect weight loss program, it is necessary to find out what exercises are perfect for you. There are as many advocates of free weights as there are of gyms and machines. I suggest that you try out both and find out what suits you the best.

For some people, machines give a better shape to their body and better posture than free weights. For others, the machines just bind them down.

I would just suggest a pair of adjustable dumbbells and a bench if you want to go for free weights. Alternatively, you can use the nearest gym. Also, there are effective exercises possible that do not require you to use any machines. You can use your bodyweight as resistance for these exercises and get good results.

Exercise Routine

You should regularly do some exercises for both your upper and lower body (total body exercises). Exercises that target the largest muscle mass should be done first in the routine. So exercise your legs, chest, and back first, and then follow it up with arms, shoulders, calves, and abdominal exercises.

Exercises with machines and weights need to be done under the supervision of a professionally qualified fitness consultant, because if not done properly, they can be injurious to your health. I recommend that you to have a medical checkup and consult your doctor before you start strength training.

Where to Work Out

While there are gyms on every block these days, many people prefer not to go to gyms. Gyms, especially the more popular ones, are crowded and it is not only irritating to wait for another person to finish his/her exercise set, but it also impedes your ability to get a high intensity workout.

Another common problem with gyms, especially for women, is having to bear the nauseating smell of sweat while working out in the same gym as men. What you could do in such cases is to find a smaller gym, or one meant just for women. There are also gyms that have special times or days allocated for women. Another tip is to avoid the most popular workout places that have a swimming pool, a spa, a parlor and so on.

Though it may be outside of your comfort zone, I do suggest that you go to the gym in the beginning, as it has a variety of equipment that you will not have access to at home. Once you learn various techniques and decide what type of exercise you like, you can set up your own home gym.

Using Body Weight as Resistance

What happens if you do not have a good gym nearby or the cash to afford a gym membership? You can always use your body weight as resistance to strength train.

Some exercises that you can do without expensive equipment are as follows (feel free to Google these for video demonstrations):

Lunge: Stand with your hands on your hips and take a long step forward. Planting your foot and bending the knee while keeping your left leg behind, push off your foot, returning to the starting position until you can't do it again. Keep your chest up and back flat to avoid curving of the back.

Sissy Squat: Hold upright with one hand and keep your waist straight. Bend at your knees and lean back as far as possible and come up on your toes. Pause briefly at the lowest position and come up to the starting position slowly.

Push Up: In the regular push up position, lower yourself stretching and come up again after pausing for a while. When you can do 15 repetitions, do the same with your legs on the bed. This makes the exercise harder and force fewer repetitions, allowing more progress.

Towel Row: Roll a towel and grab it with both hands. Then looping this on to a door knob, slide your grip to the end of the towels and move your feet near the door. Lean back into a squatting position so as to stretch the back muscles. Now, pull yourself forward to exercise your last.

Towel Lateral Raise: Hold the ends of a towel about 2 feet apart and pull with one hand on your side while resisting with the other hand like the dumbbell exercise. On hitting your max rep, do the same with the other hand.

Chair Dip: Place 2 chairs facing each other and sit on one with hands on your sides and a steady grip on the chair. Place your feet on the other chair. Lower yourself by bending your elbows and be in the position till you feel a strong stretch in your chest. Reverse back to the original position and contract your triceps.

Stair Calf Raise: Stand with your feet on a step of stairs and lower your heels into a bottom stretched position. Now lift up trying to stand on your toes while keeping the knees straight. Pause for the calves to contract and go back down. When you can manage 20 repetitions, of both legs, try a one legged calf raise which makes things harder.

Reverse Crunch: Lie on the floor and place your arms on the side. Bend your legs slightly at the knees. Push your arms and hands against the floor and use your abdominals to curl the legs and hips up and off the floor. Pause and return to the original position until you can do no more.

If you are using your bodyweight as resistance, it is difficult to prescribe any particular number of repetitions or sets for the exercises, so just go until you can do no more, while still using the proper form. Doing fewer reps with the correct form is more effective than doing more with sloppy form. Plus, it will keep you from injuring yourself, which means you will be able to stay with your routine.

Cycling

You can use a stationary bike if you have it, or a real bicycle, if the weather is fine enough for a ride. Choose a route that is easy on the knees and back.

Gradual slopes and gentle hills are good, especially if the spiders use your bike more often than you do. If you go at a moderate pace, you should cycle out about 3 miles before coming back.

That should be about 30 minutes' worth of steady cycling. Don't forget to bring along water.

Walking

You can double up with this activity if you have a dog. Go for a brisk walk for about a mile—you can do this in about 20 minutes if you're in moderately good health – before coming back. If your dog needs to do some business, don't stop moving. Walk in place while waiting.

If you don't like to go out, and you have a treadmill, that's fine. If you don't have that, you can probably walk around in your house or backyard but it probably won't be much of a workout. There will always be a lot of distractions i.e. some weeds sticking out, some books to put away, etc. You might be better off with a jump rope if you want to stay indoors.

Swimming

If you have access to a pool, swimming is the best type of exercise to set your heart pumping Of course, you won't notice if you sweat, but that's okay.

It's a good workout that doesn't put strain on your joints and back. But make sure you don't just splash around.

Do slow, steady laps for at least 30 minutes, taking brief rest periods when you get tired? While you may not seem to be sweating, you are still releasing toxins through your skin and every time you breathe out.

Exercise video

And of course, you can always turn to those exercise videos you bought for window dressing. Any physical activity will help as long as they don't involve too much high impact moves and contortionism.

All exercise videos have at least one section that uses aerobic exercises. Concentrate on these and if you have to, loop it to squeeze at least 30 minutes of activity.

It's much like dancing, but you'll feel less ridiculous following a routine on television than dancing by yourself.

How Exercising Helps You Lose Weight

Should you go for either diets or exercises in order to lose weight? This is a predicament many face when they are trying to lose weight. Escalating the confusion is that there is a lot of contradicting advice on the subject. But the truth is that both of these are needed. However, dieting is what comes first.

Think about it, if you eat more than what your body requires, it means you will have extra calories that will, in the end, cause weight gain. So you must ensure that you reduce your calorie intake.

Your goal is to eat fewer calories than what your body needs.

However, cutting calories alone is not enough. And that is where physical activity comes in. For example, if you reduce calorie intake by 500 and use another 500 calories in a workout, you will be able to lose 2 pounds in 7 days (remember that 3500 calories make 1 pound).

Furthermore, when you reach your desired weight, exercising will keep it from climbing back up.

Other benefits of Working Out

The best part with exercising is that it is not only good for your weight as it also improves your overall life.

Reduces Risk of Heart Attack - This is one of the leading causes of death. But if you exercise, you can reduce your chances of suffering from a heart attack.

Get in Shape - Although some people are born with great looking bodies, some need to work for them through exercises. In the end, not only will you be proud of your body, but you will also increase your confidence.

Improves Your Mood - If you are feeling stressed, 30 minutes per day in the gym is all you need to wash away all your worries.

There are other benefits you will get just by exercising, these are just a few.

Important Things to Remember When Exercising

Sometimes, despite spending hours on the treadmill, you may still not lose as much weight as you thought you would. What you may not know is that you could be ignoring some important things during your workouts.

So here they are:

Vary Your Workouts – Your body is very smart. When working out, it will try to find ways of making the exercise easy. So with time, it will adapt, and yes, the exercise will start feeling like a walk in the park. Unfortunately, that means you will require less effort to do the same workout. As a result, you will be using fewer calories than before.

In response, you must ensure that you vary your workouts from time to time. For example, you can run for two weeks, then swim for another two weeks. Or else, you can try mixing different workouts throughout the week.

If you do that, your body will not adapt and you will still be using more energy during each exercise.

Don't Waste Time with Breaks – The problem with many people when exercising is that they take breaks that are too long. But this is a mistake. It kills momentum and reduces your metabolic rate thereby slashing your chances of losing weight fast.

Understand that intensity is what brings results. So try to keep your breaks as brief as possible. Your focus should be to get to the finish line as fast as you can.

Listen to Music – I don't know about you, but I cannot exercise without some beats banging in my ears. When you have the right music, you force your body to not listen to how tired you are. Instead, it concentrates on how great it feels to move to the beat. This enhances your performance and it is the reason you will find music in most gyms.

The trick, however, is to have the right music. If your playlist is too slow, you won't see much improvement in your workouts.

Have a Buddy – If you find it hard to stay on an exercise routine, even after using music, you will need to find a friend who also wants to lose weight. By exercising with her you will push each other when you start feeling weak.

As a precaution, make sure you share the same goals with your friend. Otherwise, you will want to run when she wants to bench press.

Don't Forget to Warm-Up – Warming up before you start exercising is very important. It gets your muscles ready for the workouts you plan on doing. If you skimp on warming up, your muscles will be cold limiting your ability to use your body. Additionally, you risk injuring yourself.

So before you start exercising, warm-up; 5-10 minutes is all you need.

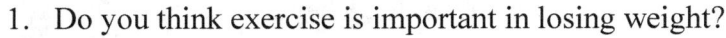

Checklist 9

1. Do you think exercise is important in losing weight?

A. Yes

B. Somewhat

C. Unsure

D. Not at all

2. Do you do any of the said activities in this chapter?

A. Yes

B. Somewhat

C. Unsure

D. Not at all

3. Do you do warm ups before exercise?

A. Yes

B. Somewhat

C. Unsure

D. Not at all

4. Do you listen to music when doing your work out?

A. Yes

B. Somewhat

C. Unsure

D. Not at all

5. Do you vary your workouts?

A. Yes

B. Somewhat

C. Unsure

D. Not at all

6. Do you think exercise helps you to improve your mood?

A. Yes

B. Somewhat

C. Unsure

D. Not at all

Do you feel that exercise helps you to improve your overall health?

A. Yes

B. Somewhat

C. Unsure

D. Not at all

Chapter 10:

Maintaining the weight loss

Losing weight is complicated. Although the diets and exercises given in this book are enough to make you shed some pounds, sometimes, these two may not bring the change you want to see.

As part of planning a maintenance regimen, you have to make a new grocery list for food that will bring you back up to a normal, balanced diet.

You may now include meat, potatoes, coffee, sugar, and all the other food items that were eliminated from your diet.

But to attain your ideal weight, you should continue to avoid food that are high in fat, sugar and bad carbohydrates as well as other bad habits, such as skipping meals and sleeping late. A list of food to avoid includes:

Fried foods

Food high in fat

Fast food and high fat snack foods

Rich gravies and sauces

Alcoholic drinks, sodas, sweetened beverages

Sugar

White bread and crackers

You should also continue doing aerobic exercises at least 3 times a week, one hour a day. You have no need to do increments at this point.

If you have comfortably worked your way up to one hour in the program, then that's fine. But if you still feel too winded, drop down to a time period that you are more comfortable with and increase it in succeeding days until you reach one hour of sustained activity.

All of the detoxifying activities describe in this program can be used on a daily basis, save for the detox drink.

You may safely go on a similar detoxification program every six months or so if you feel you need it. But if you are maintaining a healthy regimen, once a year should be more than enough.

Keep the Motivation Alive

Losing weight is complicated. Although the diets and exercises given in this book are enough to make you shed some pounds, sometimes, these two may not bring the change you want to see.

To ensure that you do not starve in vain or sweat without losing any weight, follow the tips below:

Sleep

You surely have heard that getting enough sleep is good for your health. But what you may not know is that getting some shut-eye is also important for weight loss. The problem is that if you do not get enough sleep, you wake up feeling weak. So in order to get through the day, you start reaching for other foods to give you energy. Unfortunately, this raises the number of calories in your diet.

As a remedy, make sure that you go to bed in good time. The recommendation is that you should sleep for 6-8 hours daily.

Drink Enough Water

There is no harm in drinking as much water as you can. Not only does it clean your body, but it also keeps your hunger at bay, ensuring that you do not crave other unhealthy foods. So drink 8 glasses of water daily.

The good thing is that there are no calories in water. So if you feel thirsty, you are definitely not drinking enough.

Fight Stress

As said earlier, stress slows your metabolism. But at the same time, it also increases the risk of binge eating. So train yourself to realize when you are feeling stressed. Once you do, take measures to eliminate the cause.

Watch Portion Sizes

There is no excuse for eating more food than you need even if it is low in calories. So every time when filling your plate, take only what you need. If you ignore this, you will be ingesting more food, which may later lead to an increase in weight.

Get Rid of Junk Food

You can make a promise that you will resist any food in the house that is not healthy. However, that is easy to say. It's only when you are face to face with the junk foods that you realize how difficult it is to keep your promise. So do yourself a favor; get rid of all junk food.

Consult Your Doctor

If you have a certain condition, I recommend that you consult your doctor before you start following any advice in this book or use any of the diets that I recommended. Some diets cut too many calories which make them dangerous to people with some conditions. Remember the old saying that it is better to be safe than sorry.

Now that you have enough weapons on your belt to make a change, the next thing that you need to do is to make sure that you can make it last. Unfortunately, this is a hard thing to do and this only leads people to get back into the cycle of binge eating.

Keep a picture of your old self

Sometimes, a look back is all you need in order to keep pushing forward. Once you get rid of binge eating, you will notice the difference it has made on your physical, psychological and emotional state. This becomes your new self.

However, it is very easy to get lost in your new self and slip into your old habits. Once you get that feeling that you're getting back into your old ways, just remember the pain you've suffered before your success. If possible, look at a picture of your old self and feel the resentment of ever going back to that state. Sometimes, this resentment is enough to keep you disciplined.

Seek support

Two is always better than one. Knowing that you have some people behind your back as you go into a battle between overeating and healthy eating can already help a lot. Make sure that you get enough support from your family and friends. They will be the ones to pat your back whenever you needed one.

Think of your hard work

More than dwelling on the fact that you are now better, you should concentrate on the hard work involved in getting there. Thinking of the hurdles and challenges along the way can make you feel proud, but it can also make you feel more relaxed to the point of laziness. Remember that hard work must be consistent and must not stop at any point.

Allow room for mistakes

There will be times when you will find yourself making a mistake by binge eating once in a while. Don't be too conscious about this, otherwise you'd be giving much attention to your mistake rather than your success. Making mistakes is only normal, so always allow some room for you to mess up. However, do not make a mistake twice in a row. Once you made a mistake, make sure to make no excuses except that it is normal and part of the healing process. After that, get back on track and forget about your mistake.

Reward yourself without food

The most important part of motivation is the reward. Just remember that this time around, it will not be food. Rewards are what you get and look forward to for having worked hard the entire week or month. Failure to reward yourself can make you feel deprived, so it a must to keep the motivation alive.

Checklist 10

1. Do you think maintaining your weight said in this chapter is applicable to you?

A. Yes

B. Somewhat

C. Unsure

D. Not at all

2. Do you think enough sleep is necessary in maintaining your weight?

A. Yes

B. Somewhat

C. Unsure

D. Not at all

3. Do you think stress has a great contribution in gaining weight?

A. Yes

B. Somewhat

C. Unsure

D. Not at all

4. Do you think water therapy is effective in losing weight?

A. Yes

B. Somewhat

C. Unsure

D. Not at all

5. Do you watch portion sizes of the food you take?

A. Yes

B. Somewhat

C. Unsure

D. Not at all

Do you think medical help is necessary in losing weight especially in women?

A. Yes

B. Somewhat

C. Unsure

D. Not at all

Do you receive support from your family and friends in your endeavour on losing weight?

A. Yes

B. Somewhat

C. Unsure

D. Not at all

Conclusion

When you are a woman, weight loss ultimately requires a healthy combination of good food and proper exercise. If you can find innovative and creative ways to sustain your motivation enough to establish a healthy lifestyle. You will soon find yourself losing weight at a rapid pace, without having to undergo punishing workouts or depriving diets. Eat healthy foods that provide you with enough energy to get through the day, and work out in such a manner that you are not left lifeless at the end of the day.

You should enjoy your routine so that you do not dread waking up in the mornings. Slowly start incorporating various healthy parts of the new lifestyle into your existing lifestyle, so that you are not shocked or let down by all the healthy choices you need to make to shed that extra weight. Most important of all, do not give up! Stick with the choices for long enough and you will soon accept them into your life wholeheartedly.